Praise for *Rethinking Your Unit Council Structure*

"Finally, a practical and useful tool for point-of-service professional governance leaders looking to make a difference in their profession and their practice. This book serves as a concise, applicable guide to good council decision-making and successful processes associated with effective unit council work. I strongly recommend it as the handbook for all council members and professional governance leaders."

–Tim Porter-O'Grady, DM, EdD, APRN, FAAN, FACCWS
Senior Partner, Health Systems, TPOG Associates, Inc.
Clinical Professor, School of Nursing, Emory University
Board Chair, American Nurses Foundation
Board Certified Clinical Wound Specialist

"The FLIGHT Model shatters the glass! Finally, a fresh and innovative approach that flips conventional unit-based governance on its head. The FLIGHT Model breaks through professional silos, fully engages our multigenerational workforce, celebrates creativity and innovation, and, most importantly, addresses the challenge of participation in governance—the fundamental reason many unit-based approaches suffer. I have seen the model in action, and it is thrilling—read this book!"

–Celia Guarino, MSN, RN, NEA-BC
Chief Nursing Officer
Holy Cross Health & Holy Cross Hospital

"The authors of this book have expertly outlined a unit-level decision-making process that ultimately improves outcomes. Bravo! Shared governance councils should do just that. This book describes a variation in the traditional model that exemplifies the creativity of organizations to make meaningful unit-level decisions for their teams. Kudos to the risk-taking leaders and clinical staff who brought this innovation to life and to the authors for sharing their success with the healthcare world."

–Marky Medeiros, MSN, RN
Consultant, Creative Health Care Management
Coauthor, *Shared Governance That Works*

RETHINKING YOUR
UNIT COUNCIL
STRUCTURE

an innovative approach to professional governance in healthcare

Beth Browder, MHSA, BSN, RN-BC, NE-BC
Gilbert Fuentes, MSN, RN, CMSRN, ONC
Roxanne Holm, MSN, RN-BC
Deborah Macy, BSN, RN-BC
Jacqui Middlemiss, BSN, RN, ONC, CMSRN

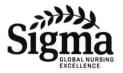

Sigma
GLOBAL NURSING
EXCELLENCE

The Sigma Theta Tau International Honor Society of Nursing (Sigma) is a nonprofit organization whose mission is advancing world health and celebrating nursing excellence in scholarship, leadership, and service. Founded in 1922, Sigma has more than 135,000 active members in over 90 countries and territories. Members include practicing nurses, instructors, researchers, policymakers, entrepreneurs, and others. Sigma's more than 530 chapters are located at more than 700 institutions of higher education throughout Armenia, Australia, Botswana, Brazil, Canada, Colombia, England, Ghana, Hong Kong, Ireland, Japan, Jordan, Kenya, Lebanon, Malawi, Mexico, the Netherlands, Nigeria, Pakistan, the Philippines, Portugal, Puerto Rico, Singapore, South Africa, South Korea, Swaziland, Sweden, Taiwan, Tanzania, Thailand, the United States, and Wales. Learn more at www.sigmanursing.org.

Sigma Theta Tau International
550 West North Street
Indianapolis, IN, USA 46202

To order additional books, buy in bulk, or order for corporate use, contact Sigma Marketplace at 888.654.4968 (US and Canada) or +1.317.634.8171 (outside US and Canada).

To request a review copy for course adoption, email solutions@sigmamarketplace.org or call 888.654.4968 (US and Canada) or +1.317.634.8171 (outside US and Canada).

To request author information, or for speaker or other media requests, contact Sigma Marketing at 888.634.7575 (US and Canada) or +1.317.634.8171 (outside US and Canada).

ISBN: 9781945157943
EPUB ISBN: 9781945157950
PDF ISBN: 9781945157967
MOBI ISBN: 9781945157974

Library of Congress Cataloging-in-Publication data

Names: Browder, Beth, 1962- author. | Fuentes, Gilbert, 1985- author. | Holm,
 Roxanne, 1970- author. | Macy, Deborah, author. | Middlemiss, Jacqui,
 author. | Sigma Theta Tau International, issuing body.
Title: Rethinking your unit council structure : an innovative approach to
 professional governance in healthcare / Beth Browder, Gilbert Fuentes, Roxanne
 Holm, Deborah Macy, Jacqui Middlemiss.
Description: Indianapolis, IN, USA : Sigma Theta Tau International, [2019] |
 Includes bibliographical references.
Identifiers: LCCN 2019016636| ISBN 9781945157943 (print) | ISBN 9781945157950
 (epub) | ISBN 9781945157967 (pdf) | ISBN 9781945157974 (mobi)
Subjects: | MESH: Shared Governance, Nursing--methods | Nursing
 Staff--organization & administration | Leadership | Decision Making,
 Organizational
Classification: LCC RT89 | NLM WY 105 | DDC 362.17/3068--dc23 LC record available at
 https://lccn.loc.gov/2019016636

First Printing, 2019

Publisher: Dustin Sullivan
Acquiring Editor: Emily Hatch
Publications Specialist: Todd Lothery
Cover Designer: Rebecca Batchelor
Interior Design/Page Layout: Rebecca Batchelor

Managing Editor: Carla Hall
Development and Project Editor: Meaghan O'Keeffe
Copy Editor: Erin Geile
Proofreader: Gill Editorial Services
Indexer: Larry D. Sweazy

Dedications

This book is dedicated to all nurses who strive to create positive change in their workplace—those nurses who recognize opportunities to improve the lives of both their colleagues and their patients and who go above and beyond to implement change.

Additionally, we dedicate this book to all the members of our healthcare teams that have been involved in our transformative journey to create an improved unit council structure—specifically, the clinical nurses and nurse leaders who were unit council chairs and coaches at the time our story began.

Finally, we would like to dedicate this book to the entire unit council team at John Muir Health: the nurses, nursing assistants, secretaries, physical therapists, occupational therapists, dieticians, pharmacists, respiratory therapists, physicians, and educators. You are the reason this new unit council structure has been successful. You saw an opportunity, and you weren't afraid to jump in and solve problems. You rallied to identify best practices and have continued to work tirelessly to implement a better approach. We wouldn't be here without all of you.

Thank you.

Acknowledgments

Life is crazy—we are proof of that. One day, a group of nurses decided there was a problem that needed fixing. Before you know it, that same group was asked to write a book. That group was us. We all eagerly said, "You bet!" None of us had written a book before, and we naively thought it would be easy enough to do. We were wrong. Although writing this book has been more challenging than we thought, it has also been an experience we will never forget. The bonds we have made as colleagues and now friends, the tears of frustration and tears of joy we shed, and the respect for the writing process we uncovered are profound.

This adventure could not have happened without the unwavering support of our spouses. Their willingness to accept our crazy work and writing schedules, their culinary skills, and their devotion to supporting our success was, without exception, magnificent. They kept life going while we hunkered down to work. Most importantly, they bought us wine.

While our spouses supported our efforts, our children (and grandchildren) provided us with balance and meaning. In each "book club" session, at least one, if not all, of our children were discussed. Our children range in age from 2 to 36. We had a lot to talk about. Mostly, we had a lot to laugh about.

We cannot forget our parents. We appreciate your support cheering us on at childhood sporting events, music recitals, school plays, road trips, sleepovers, and so many other events, and we wouldn't have gotten where we needed to be without your taxi service. We may have outgrown our childhood stuffed animals, but we will never outgrow needing your love and support in our adulthood. Your continued support is evidenced through your attendance at the 2017 Magnet conference—sitting in the front row (and taking us out to dinner that night) to listen to us tell our story over and over (and over, again) as we figured out our words. Your ongoing pride in our accomplishments and your welcoming hugs warm our hearts. We are as proud of you as you are of us.

We also give thanks to our work families at John Muir Health. All of us work with different teams, and they have cheered us from the sidelines, at times given us much needed encouragement, and helped craft a work schedule that allowed time for writing. Our fellow nurses provided us with inspiration, vision, and purpose. Specifically, we acknowledge Michelle Lopes, System Chief

Nurse Executive, for listening to and validating our change proposal and for realizing the important work that clinical nurses do at the bedside. We thank Vivian Brailoff, Program Manager for Magnet, who wrote our abstract that was eventually accepted for podium presentation at the 2017 Magnet conference. It was at this conference that Sigma heard our presentation and approached us about a book. Without Vivian, you literally would not be reading our book. We appreciate and thank Molly Tappe, Professional Development Specialist, for the hours and hours she spent swimming in data and helping us to define whether our change was impactful. She works tirelessly with many groups to help quantify outcomes. Bless her. We honor Onette Krigbaum, Coordinator of Professional Practice and Shared Governance, who is the glue for all of us. She is warm, funny, spunky, and ready to fight real and imagined dragons for us. And we thank Nancy Gibbs, Professional Development Specialist, who was undoubtedly our biggest cheerleader. She inspired us to be our best, to try, and to soar. She sat in the front row of our podium presentation and cheered like a proud mom at a tennis match.

We would be remiss if we did not give a huge shout-out to everyone who contributed their ideas and inspiration to this project. This includes both past and present unit council chairs and coaches who were willing to risk it all to find a new way. It also includes the dedicated and hardworking nurses who formed our unit council redesign work group. They were fearless and willing to put it all on the line to forge a future that would be relevant and meaningful. Were it not for this group, the status quo would have prevailed.

We acknowledge the American Nurses Credentialing Center and the Magnet program office as well. Without them, our presentation might never have materialized. Thank you for allowing us to present our story at the Magnet conference in Houston, Texas, in 2017. Imagine our shock when we learned we would be presenting to an audience of over 1,300 participants. When our nerves settled, we realized that we had, in fact, been given a gift. The audience members talked to us long after our presentation concluded, and we felt a deep common bond as nurses pursuing best practice and supporting a culture of excellence. We have always been proud to be nurses, but we were especially proud that day.

Finally, we are grateful and humble for Sigma's publishing team. Emily Hatch, Acquiring Book Editor, heard our presentation, found value in the information, and saw potential for a book. We never, not even once, thought about a book. Because of her encouraging approach, we began to think differently.

Emily believed in us and guided us in our journey as first-time authors. We are grateful to Meaghan O'Keeffe, Development and Project Editor, who took our manuscript and made it much, much better. You are amazing and a gift to the world. We are indebted to the entire Sigma publishing team. What you do behind the scenes should be shouted from the rooftops.

Finally, we are grateful for each other. What a crazy life!

About the Authors*

Beth Browder, MHSA, BSN, RN-BC, NE-BC: Beth Browder has been a nurse for over 30 years and has been in leadership roles for the last 20 years. She is currently Executive Director for Professional Nursing Practice, Quality, and Education and the Magnet Program Director for John Muir Health. She holds a BSN from Washburn University in Topeka, Kansas, and a master's in health services administration from the University of Kansas in Kansas City, Kansas. Browder has experience in behavioral health, legal nurse consulting, utilization review, hospice, case management, clinical education, and quality improvement. She has worked in a variety of organizations and has developed, implemented, and revised nursing governance processes at each organization. She is a strong proponent of professional governance concepts and uses every opportunity to help others be successful in their endeavors with maintaining a governance structure—even in times of lean financial operations and cost-cutting initiatives.

Gilbert Fuentes, MSN, RN, CMSRN, ONC: Gilbert Fuentes is a certified medical-surgical and orthopedic nursing leader with more than 10 years of acute care experience. He holds an ADN from College of the Redwoods, a BSN from California State University, East Bay, and an MSN from the University of Arizona. He has extensive leadership experience in developing projects that improve patient outcomes, patient care, and employee engagement on both unit and system levels. For many years, he has been a designated unit level council coach and a liaison to the systemwide unit council committee. In his daily work he uses transformational leadership and innovative techniques to design unit level and systemwide projects that improve quality outcomes and employee satisfaction.

Roxanne Holm, MSN, RN-BC: Roxanne Holm has been a nurse for 25 years and has held various positions and cared for diverse patient populations. Throughout her career she has worked on creating work environments where the bedside nurse can be a change agent through professional governance. Her most recent focus is supporting the unit council structure and providing the knowledge and opportunities necessary for unit council success. She is currently a Nursing Professional Development Specialist in Acute Care and is a certified professional development specialist. She holds a BSN from the University of Iowa and an MSN in nursing administration from the University of Nebraska Medical Center.

Deborah Macy, BSN, RN-BC: Deborah Macy is a Unit Supervisor on a medical-surgical unit that specializes in endocrine, renal, and stroke patient populations at John Muir Health. As a supervisor, she is responsible for clinical practice and employee education to maintain quality standards of care for the population served. Macy holds a BSN and is working toward her MSN in nursing education. She has over 30 years of practice in the acute care setting. She maintains specialty certification in medical-surgical nursing through the American Nurses Association. Her leadership experience includes being a Unit Supervisor and a BSN Clinical Instructor. She serves as the unit council coach and was coach as the organization developed and implemented the new unit council structure with the FLIGHT Model.

Jacqui Middlemiss, BSN, RN, ONC, CMSRN: Jacqui Middlemiss has over 10 years of nursing experience with specialty certification in orthopedic nursing and medical-surgical nursing. She holds a BSN from Sonoma State University and currently works as a clinical nurse and relief charge nurse on an endocrine, renal, and stroke unit at John Muir Health. She is a strong patient advocate and has been involved with many performance improvement projects surrounding patient care and increasing employee and patient satisfaction. Middlemiss has served as her unit council's chair when she had the idea for a new unit council structure; she was also a member of the work group to develop and implement the new structure. Recognized as her organization's Magnet Nurse of the Year in 2017, she is passionate about creating and embracing change and empowering others to do the same.

All the authors are local and national speakers on the FLIGHT Model for unit-based professional governance.

Contents

APPENDIXES

FOREWORD

It is my sincerest honor and privilege to write the foreword for *Rethinking Your Unit Council Structure: An Innovative Approach to Professional Governance in Healthcare*. As the System Chief Nurse Executive working with the authors—a phenomenal team of professional nurses—on this innovative unit council model, I am proud to introduce their collaborative work.

Over the course of my career I have participated in unit-based governance as both a staff nurse and a leader. Years ago, I remember a fellow leader telling me, "If you need to solve a problem at the bedside, get the unit-based professional nurses together, give them the resources they need, and then get out of their way." In my years as a nursing leader, I have seen this phenomenon play out time after time. As a result, I am a fierce advocate of professional governance.

When I began as a new graduate nurse many years ago, we did things the way we were taught and did not question otherwise—a hard practice to break anywhere. And then came one of the most exciting problem-solving evolutions that I have seen in my career: the FLIGHT Model. I have such a powerful memory of the first time I heard about this new idea for our unit-based councils. We had struggled for years with generating energy and adequate participation on our councils, until one day, an exceptional bedside nurse asked the question: "What if?" And from that one question and that one idea, the transformation of our professional governance unit-based council structure was born!

The FLIGHT Model, as presented in this book, highlights an approach that is professionally designed, outcome-focused, interprofessional, and absolutely genius! It is an approach that makes me excited to be a nurse, proud to be a leader, and inspired to work alongside such innovative, accomplished nurses. I did not come up with this model, but I fully support it and encourage those who are struggling with their unit-based governance structure to consider adopting it. You will not be disappointed.

I'd like to thank the exceptional nurses and authors of this book for their dedication to our organization, their passion for the nursing profession, and their commitment to the innovative evolution of professional governance. Each one of you inspires me to be a better leader and supporter of those at the front lines of patient care—nurses who give more to our patients and their families than we could ever ask for.

–Michelle Lopes, MSN, RN, NEA-BC
Senior Vice President, Chief Nurse Executive
John Muir Health

INTRODUCTION

"There's a way to do it better—find it!"

–Thomas A. Edison

When problems arise, opportunity exists for creative solutions. Most people, however, have trouble viewing change positively. As you read this book, think about the gifts and strengths of the people on your team and who can best help you achieve successful results. You will need to surround yourself with colleagues who can embrace change and feel energized and excited about the prospect of creating positive outcomes. We were able to make it happen, and so can you.

We found that the unit council structures typically found in the clinical arena struggled to keep up with the rapid changes occurring in healthcare today. The FLIGHT Model of unit-based professional governance was developed by a group of registered nurses working in a large community hospital in the East Bay area of California. The model was developed out of frustration. These registered nurses, in varying levels of leadership at their organization, came to the realization that the traditional model of unit council was no longer meeting the needs of the organization, the nurses working on the units, or the inter-professional team members they worked alongside. They wanted to make a change in the organization at the unit level—but competing forces, budgetary restrictions, and the way in which councils were organized hindered the ability of many councils to be successful. The overwhelming frustration felt by these nurses is summarized in the words of a unit council chair: "There *must* be a better way." The FLIGHT Model is that better way.

The FLIGHT Model stands for Fostering Leadership, Innovation, and Growth through Healthcare Teams; it is a framework within which a team can achieve the ideals of professional governance. It empowers the entire interprofessional team to develop and implement change to improve patient care, influence professional development, and promote collaboration among the care team. Projects developed within the FLIGHT Model connect and unite team members toward achieving overarching organizational goals. Momentum remains as leadership and clinical employee move together toward a unified destination. While there may be the occasional change in flight plan or unexpected turbulence, all are working together toward the ultimate organizational destination.

Because of the limitations and frustrations felt under the traditional unit council structure, we experienced an increase in burnout among unit council members. A commitment of two years was required to be a part of the council, and typically each unit contained 8 to 10 members at one time. The challenges faced by the unit council members made it difficult to recruit new members. There have been many studies over the years regarding stress and burnout among healthcare professionals. As Laschinger and Leiter note, "A major source of burnout is an overloaded work schedule, that is, having too little time and too few resources to accomplish the job. Lack of control, performing tasks that conflict with employee values and beliefs, and a breakdown in social work factors are also factors that lead to burnout" (2006, p. 260). The members on each unit council were being asked to complete projects that did not always affect them, and they were not necessarily passionate about every topic or project they worked on. Perhaps it was a request from the manager to improve workflow on the unit or responding to complaints from employees and being responsible for "fixing" those problems. One can imagine how these council members became overwhelmed with the demands and sometimes lacked the recognition they deserved.

Havens, Gittell, and Vasey (2018) define *relational coordination* as "a mutually reinforcing process of communication and relating for the purpose of task integration" (p. 133). In their recent study, they compared relational coordination with nurse job satisfaction, work engagement, and burnout. They determined that there was a consistent relationship between relational coordination and nurse reports of well-being. "This finding is highly relevant, given current concerns about healthcare provider burnout, morale, and general well-being" and plays an important role in navigating ways to improve the interprofessional experience (Havens et al., 2018, p. 137). Initiatives such as "selecting providers for teamwork, measuring team performance, resolving conflicts proactively, investing in frontline leadership, developing shared protocols, broadening participation in team meetings and developing shared information systems" can go a long way in improving employee morale and preventing burnout (Havens et al., 2018, p. 138). The identified characteristics in these studies are directly related to the development and benefits of the FLIGHT Model.

Change is continual and ongoing. When we started our journey with the FLIGHT Model, the terminology used was *shared governance*. A shift toward *professional governance* is taking place in the literature. We embrace this changing terminology and believe it supports our vision of professional nurses working with interprofessional teams. In most instances in this book, you will find we use *professional governance* with the exception of direct quotes or situations where a historical perspective is better served with *shared governance*.

The next sections describe our journey and the genesis for developing the FLIGHT Model. We are certain you will be able to identify with our struggles but also see that there is hope for an engaged, outcome-focused, and collegial employee-driven option.

Our Story

Something Amiss

Jacqui, a unit council chair on a busy 34-bed medical unit, realized a need for change within her council. Members vacillated from being engaged to essentially being absent. The council projects progressed slowly and felt never-ending, and there was a lack of energy and support from the general unit team members. When networking with other unit council chairs, Jacqui learned that many others felt similarly.

One day, Deborah, a supervisor on Jacqui's unit, sent a unit-wide email soliciting employee interest in forming a small task force. The email outlined the task force's role—to review a specific workflow proposal that a clinical nurse had learned at a recent nursing conference and determine feasibility of implementing this new practice. Jacqui responded with interest and was selected to join the work group, which included other nurses who weren't currently involved in the unit council. As the task force began to work on the proposal, Jacqui noticed a tremendous amount of energy and excitement. Various disciplines were involved in the task force and appeared highly engaged in contributing—something she rarely saw in her unit council projects. Jacqui attributed this energy to their desire to be involved in this project and that the team was eager to make a change on an issue they were passionate about. Every member felt inspired and empowered to contribute toward a positive change.

Jacqui began to question the current, traditional way of her unit council structure. Some of her questions included:

- What if this kind of energy and engagement were seen with unit council projects?
- Why is our unit council having so much difficulty when there are clearly people working on the unit who are passionate about creating change?

- Is the current structure too rigid? If so, what if we created a more flexible and inclusive environment?
- Would more people be willing to share their ideas and work on a project if it didn't involve an extended time commitment?
- There are so many employees on each unit—why are we limiting our council to a finite number of members?

When networking with chairs from other departments, Jacqui shared her experience with being a member of the interprofessional task force on her unit. She shared with these chairs the difference in engagement, enthusiasm, and ownership of the work she witnessed as compared to her own unit council.

Between her conversations with other unit council chairs and more self-reflection, Jacqui realized she had additional questions:

- What if employees came up with ideas and felt empowered to bring forth solutions?
- What if the employee who had the solution was the person in charge of the project?
- What if they could ask others interested in the project to work collaboratively, thus being more flexible, fluid, and inclusive?

In addition to her observations, a survey of all unit council chairs had been conducted three months prior. According to this survey, the top three areas where unit council chairs struggled were:

- Recruiting new members
- Managing projects
- Using evidence-based practice to guide projects

A New Vision

These questions and the results of the survey began to congeal, and the beginnings of a concept emerged. Jacqui wanted a process that would engage more employees and tap into individual talents and interests. She felt her concept could potentially address many of the problems the councils had long been facing.

Approximately every other month, the chairs and coaches of all unit councils meet as a group. Jacqui used this meeting to share her thoughts and rough concept regarding a need to find a new way. Roxanne, a clinical educator and the facilitator of this meeting, encouraged Jacqui to meet with the Director of Professional Practice and share her idea.

Jacqui and Deborah (the unit council coach) met with Beth, Director of Professional Practice, Quality, and Safety. They shared Jacqui's innovative idea and her thoughts about a more inclusive and flexible environment where employees could feel empowered to create and lead change. Jacqui shared her vision and the thought process that evolved. To Jacqui's relief, Beth was supportive of this new and innovative concept. The excitement and energy were palpable as this small group became infused with hope. Because of organizational initiatives, Beth realized the window of opportunity for this change was very narrow and encouraged immediately forming a work group to brainstorm and flesh out a new structure.

Change is difficult. The same unit council structure had been in place for almost 10 years. Clinical nurses and nursing leaders knew what to expect of the unit council process and were comfortable with it—even though it wasn't working. As is typical with any type of change, doubts immediately began to surface, and there were reservations when the idea was brought back to the unit council leader group. However, because there was enough evidence of lack of employee engagement, frustration, and the general sense that something had to change, the decision was made to move forward. Rather than looking back at how it had once been, it was time to start building a new council structure.

A work group was formed to envision an ideal unit council structure. The work group identified a gap between organizational priorities and malalignment with unit council projects. They knew this needed to be addressed or unit council work would not have the needed organizational support to be successful. To help this process, they envisioned three focus areas that unit council projects should align:

- Patient satisfaction/engagement
- Employee satisfaction/engagement
- Quality and safety improvements

They found a second gap in quantifying improvements. In the previous structure, there were great projects, but they were not structured to include pre- and post-project improvement metrics. It was realized that more focus on measuring the results of change and developing evidence was necessary. Projects would no longer be based primarily on employee complaints, but rather on consistently using data in a more efficient way to show outcome improvements.

The last gap that we identified was the composition of a unit council. The work group agreed the new unit council structure would focus on the entire unit as the council—and not an identified group of nurses as seen in the past. They wanted every employee member to have the opportunity to create a project, join in on a project, lead a project, and feel empowered by having a voice in creating positive changes for the unit and the hospital.

This team knew they needed to develop a new model, outline new tools, and create an entirely new structure that would take months to design and implement. This was exciting yet daunting, as redesigning an entirely new unit council structure would be a new adventure. This book is the result of that work and the model that was developed.

We are so excited to share our story with you and hope that you will be able to successfully implement the FLIGHT Model into your organization, as we have done in ours.

Book Overview

Rethinking Your Unit Council Structure is divided into three parts:

Part 1: The Mechanics of FLIGHT

We set the stage for you in Chapter 1 by identifying the changing healthcare environment, including changing patient demographics, the multigenerational workforce, and the financial picture healthcare organizations face today.

In Chapter 2, we outline the history of shared governance and its importance in supporting ownership, accountability, equity, and partnership. We illustrate why the FLIGHT Model is effective and beneficial for any healthcare organization.

Part 2: Mastering Aerodynamics

Chapter 3 covers the FLIGHT Model in detail, including a visual depiction, the four pillars, and the innovative ways the model can change project flow when implemented.

Chapter 4 identifies characteristics of leadership and how the styles of leadership influence the success of professional governance and implementing the FLIGHT Model.

In Chapter 5 we discuss how to analyze the current state, envision opportunity, and engage leadership and clinical employees. This chapter helps you evaluate how effective your current state is and what your ideal state could look like.

Part 3: Taking FLIGHT

Chapter 6 outlines different change theories and their necessity in the process of transformational change. We apply John Kotter's Change Theory to the FLIGHT Model and show you how you can do the same for your organization. We provide examples, using case studies, to illustrate the different stages of change.

Chapter 7 includes the tools and training tips you need to implement the FLIGHT Model. In this chapter we provide you with everything you will need to create a successful unit council structure.

Chapter 8 covers how to maximize and sustain project results across an organization through project sharing. We recognize the importance and value of celebrating successes of all sizes, communicating that success, and encouraging others to do the same.

Throughout the book, you will find case studies that illustrate real-world examples using the FLIGHT Model, as well as tips to keep in mind while implementing changes using this innovative unit council structure.

Our Goals for This Book

It is our hope that, through this book, whether you are a clinical employee feeling encouraged to propose a new idea or create change, or you are a leader who realizes the need to improve a less-than-ideal process, you feel inspired and motivated to do so. Our desire is to provide you with the tools and evidence you need to create a successful new process for your organization.

References

Havens, D. S., Gittell, J. H., & Vasey, J. (2018). Impact of relational coordination on nurse job satisfaction, work engagement and burnout: Achieving the Quadruple Aim. *JONA: The Journal of Nursing Administration, 48*(3), 132–140. doi:10.1097/nna.0000000000000587

Laschinger, H. K., & Leiter, M. P. (2006). The impact of nursing work environments on patient safety outcomes: The mediating role of burnout/engagement. *JONA: The Journal of Nursing Administration, 36*(5), 259–267.

1

THE MECHANICS
OF FLIGHT

"We are all in some state of transition from a volume- to value-based payment system. It takes an enormous amount of resources to track and improve on hundreds of core measures and outcome metrics. Prioritizing and focusing the team on the most critical elements requires great discipline."

–Mary Lou Mastro, Elmhurst (IL) Memorial Healthcare

1

THE CHANGING FACE OF HEALTHCARE: HOW CAN WE CHANGE WITH IT?

OBJECTIVES

- Understand the financial impact of organizational decision-making
- Recognize the important role of the clinical nurse in a changing climate
- Understand the value in shifting from a discipline-specific focus toward interprofessional teamwork
- Recognize the changing faces of the healthcare employee and the patient population

It's both an exciting time and a challenging time to be in healthcare. Change is fast-paced; technology is constantly advancing. Healthcare consumers are more connected to information and resources related to their diagnosis and treatment options as well as hospital performance measures and patient outcomes. Healthcare organizations work hard to keep up with the rapid changes while striving for continual improvements. Many organizations are going through transformations, forming new partnerships, and working hard to standardize care delivery to decrease variations in practice and improve outcomes. Every employee in healthcare can play a key part in the success of their organization.

The FLIGHT Model is predicated on the notion that all members of the healthcare team have a role and a responsibility to make a difference: to improve patient care outcomes, the work environment (including their own job satisfaction), and the patient experience for those they care for on their unit. This transformative work should not be left to a small group of individuals—like those who compose a traditional unit council—but should be shared across the department, disciplines, and the organization. The FLIGHT Model encourages creativity, a team approach, and expression of individual passion by allowing interprofessional team members to be owners of projects that are important and involved in ways that fit their life. This inclusive model is in response to a quickly changing climate of healthcare, the individuality that each team member brings to the work setting, and the effectiveness of the team approach.

Influencing Forces in Healthcare

Although there are many influencing forces in the changing healthcare environment, there are a few that are worth noting for purposes of this book. They are:

- The Affordable Care Act (ACA)
- The electronic health record (EHR)
- Hospital Consumer Assessment of Healthcare Providers and Systems (HCAHPS)

The Affordable Care Act (ACA)

The ACA and an overall shift toward value-based purchasing (VBP) have been major influencers of healthcare reform in the United States, and they are requiring organizations to become high performers in quality outcomes and change the way they operate. If costs are contained and quality standards are met, organizations receive incentive payments. Conversely, if the costs or quality are not acceptable, organizational reimbursement is reduced (Medicare Learning Network, 2017). Organizations cannot afford to have poor-quality outcomes and must be continually pushing to improve. Because the VBP program is continually evolving and focusing on different measures every year, hospitals and other healthcare organizations need to be nimble and have effective teams ready and able to respond to make the necessary improvements (Dempsey, Reilly, & Buhlman, 2014). Creating sustainable practice changes to improve quality outcomes requires all members of the healthcare team to be engaged and moving in the same direction.

The Electronic Health Record (EHR)

The EHR has also changed the way care is delivered, data is pulled, and patient information is shared. Workflows, like medication administration or blood administration, now rely on technology to help prevent errors. This technology is intended to help improve patient outcomes, but it can also be cumbersome and frustrating for employees when the extra steps take more time or do not always work as envisioned (Siwicki, 2017). The EHR can also be used to extract data and trends in patient care delivery to determine if important initiatives are being successfully implemented at the point of care. Ideally, the use of EHR contributes to a safer healthcare system, but it can create new challenges for employees and requires close partnering with the organization's information technology department. These teams need to be ready to respond to ongoing changes and make timely improvements to the system, so it is more streamlined and easier to use.

The EHR is also continually being improved to support better care coordination by allowing different providers in different practice settings to work from the same database. This sharing of information reduces duplication of services and provides consistent information about prior medical care. Ideally, this database is available across the patient's care continuum. The success or failure of coordination of services can be impactful. Hospitals recognize that poor coordination can result in longer lengths of stays and delays in necessary services, which in turn, lead to poorer quality of care (Nickitas, Middaugh, & Aries, 2016).

Hospital Consumer Assessment of Healthcare Providers and Systems (HCAHPS)

Healthcare consumers influence both reimbursement and the reputations of healthcare organizations. Now, more than ever, consumers share their experiences and perspectives through surveys, social media, and other online venues. HCAHPS is a survey developed by the Centers for Medicare and Medicaid Services with the Agency for Healthcare Research and Quality and was designed for healthcare consumers to provide feedback on the following:

- Nurse communication
- Doctor communication
- Responsiveness of employees
- Pain management
- Communication about medications
- Discharge information
- Hospital environment
- Willingness to recommend
- Overall hospital rating

The results of the surveys are made available for consumers to compare how various organizations rate compared to others (Ketelsen, Cook, & Kennedy, 2014). This additional layer of transparency provides the consumer with the power of information to be more selective when making healthcare decisions. In addition, the patient experience of their services can significantly affect reimbursement. According to Dempsey et al. (2014), "Patient experience, as measured by the Hospital Consumer Assessment of Healthcare Providers and Systems (HCAHPS) survey, drives 30% of value-based purchasing (VBP) scores and incentive payments, as prescribed under the Patient Protection and Affordable Care Act" (p. 142). Even though nurses spend the most time with their patients, all healthcare employees need to be aware of the individualized needs of their patients and work hard to improve quality and the patient experience.

Within the FLIGHT Model, financial awareness, knowledge of technology, and data such as HCAHPS scores help guide unit council projects and can drive improved patient outcomes, improved organizational financial stability, and improved patient experience. The FLIGHT Model allows for all perspectives to be explored in a timely and relevant manner.

The Important Role of Nursing

According to the Bureau of Labor Statistics (2015), registered nurses make up 22.9% of healthcare employees and have the potential to be strong agents of change in healthcare. The role of the clinical nurse is central to patient care. Registered nurses are self-directed decision-makers who use theory and best practices to provide care and communicate their findings to other disciplines involved in the care of their patients. They are not only accountable to their role and the care they deliver, but they also continually monitor their practice and the outcomes associated with their interventions. It is essential that registered nurses either lead or play a role in innovative teams working to make improvements in the healthcare system (O'Rourke, 2003). Nurses are influential, important decision-makers and essential members of the interprofessional team. Organizations that focus on nurses as change agents and a valuable part of the interprofessional team understand the impact of this group of professionals.

The Future of Nursing

The world today has taken on a global perspective, and population health has the goal of providing quality healthcare to all as a basic human right. The Institute of Medicine (IOM) and the Robert Wood Johnson Foundation jointly reviewed how the nursing profession could help contribute to national concerns about delivering affordable and accessible quality healthcare to the general population. From this review, the IOM published *The Future of Nursing: Leading Change, Advancing Health* in 2010 (Battié, 2013; Committee on the Robert Wood Johnson Foundation Initiative on the Future of Nursing, Institute of Medicine, 2011).

A Note on Terminology

Change is continual and ongoing. When we started our journey with the FLIGHT Model, the terminology used was *shared governance*. A shift toward *professional governance* is taking place in the literature. We embrace this changing terminology and believe it supports our vision of professional nurses working with interprofessional teams. In most instances in this book, you will find we use *professional governance* with the exception of direct quotes or situations where a historical perspective is better served with *shared governance*.

Nurses Leading Change

One of the key messages in the IOM report focuses on the need to transform leadership. "Nurses should be full partners, with physicians and other health professionals, in redesigning health care in the United States" (Committee on the Robert Wood Johnson Foundation Initiative on the Future of Nursing, Institute of Medicine, 2011, p. 29). Nurses are at the bedside and have a direct effect on patient care. Clinical nurses may not view themselves as leaders, but they are. They work collegially together, as well as lead others in caring for their patients. They lead the patient in developing the plan of care for their health. Nursing's leadership skills contribute toward patient safety and quality of care.

IOM Report: The Future of Nursing: Leading Change, Advancing Health

"Given their direct and sustained contact with patients, front-line nurses, along with their unit or clinic managers, are uniquely positioned to design new models of care to improve quality, efficiency, and safety. Tapping that potential will require developing a new workplace culture that encourages and supports leaders at the point of care (whether a hospital or the community) and requires all members of a health care team to hold each other accountable for the team's performance; nurses must also be equipped with the communication, conflict resolution, and negotiating skills necessary to succeed in leadership and partnership roles" (Committee on the Robert Wood Johnson Foundation Initiative on the Future of Nursing, Institute of Medicine, 2011, p. 234).

In the clinical environment, clinical nurses can identify problems and areas of waste and often see a better way. These problems can be presented through complaints and can lead to statements like, "There has to be a better way to do this!" Professional governance supports clinical employees to imagine and lead a plan to address these issues. It promotes the realization and accountability that nurses help shape the healthcare system and make changes to improve patient care. Rather than policy being something that happens *to* them, they are given permission to craft policy based on best evidence. The Future of Nursing report acknowledges that "collaboration is a key strategy for improving problem solving and achieving innovation in health care" (Committee on the Robert Wood Johnson Foundation Initiative on the Future of Nursing, Institute of Medicine, 2011, p. 225).

Collaboration and engagement at all levels of an organization typifies professional governance. Through providing nurses with the opportunity to lead and providing a supported pathway to make practice changes, a successful professional governance structure allows nurses to develop necessary leadership skills and competencies to work collaboratively with other interprofessional team members.

The Power of the Interprofessional Team

Although clinical nurses are with patients 24/7 and are continually assessing the human response to various interventions, they do not work in isolation. The interprofessional team, now more than ever, must collaborate to deliver a personalized, holistic plan of care in a very complex environment. Members of the interprofessional team are driven to do the right thing but experience frustrations and challenges every day. How they handle these challenges that affect their practice can look very different throughout organizations.

In 2010, the World Health Organization (WHO) published *Framework for Action on Interprofessional Education and Collaborative Practice*. This framework is a call to action that recognizes the unique attributes of healthcare systems throughout the world and helps provide direction for how to move toward a more interprofessional approach in policymaking, decision-making, education, healthcare system design, and leadership. According to the WHO (2010), collaborative practice can:

- Improve patient outcomes
- Improve appropriate use of resources
- Improve the work environment
- Decrease the length of stay
- Decrease employee turnover
- Decrease errors
- Decrease the cost of care

There is a shift toward an interprofessional approach in healthcare; we are preparing our future workforce to value it and to have the necessary skill set to collaborate with the interprofessional team. One major focus of the WHO framework is the move toward interprofessional education. According to Gilbert, Yan, and Hoffman (2010), "interprofessional education occurs when students from two or more professions learn about, from, and with each other to enable effective collaboration and improve health outcomes" (p. 196). Incorporating interprofessional learning opportunities throughout educational programs helps create a workforce that is less disjointed and more interconnected. Starting with interprofessional education at the university level helps create a collaborative practice–ready workforce. Students training in various healthcare-related fields like physical therapy, medicine, and pharmacy have an opportunity to learn together through intentional learning activities, like simulation. Hovland, Whitford, and Niederriter (2018) studied the perspectives of nursing students following an interprofessional simulation experience. After this experience, the students believed in the power of the team and the importance of interprofessional communication, and valued working together to see the big picture around patient care. Understanding the roles, scope, and practice of the other professions helped them realize that we are better together and there is not one profession more important than another. Equity is an important principle of professional governance and should be flourishing in organizations that embrace an interprofessional model of professional governance.

The interprofessional skills learned during formal educational programs need to translate into the workplace and continuously be interwoven in educational opportunities and supported in daily workflow routines. Organizations that create opportunities for various disciplines to come together and collaborate will not only experience the benefits outlined in the WHO framework, but they will also see a transformation in their organizational culture. Having clarity of roles, mutual respect, equity, and open communication all support a coordinated approach to patient care (Bridges, Davidson, Odegard, Maki, & Tomkowiak, 2011). It is important for professionals to see themselves as a valued part of the team. Common practices like multidisciplinary rounds, interprofessional safety huddles, and interprofessional work groups create opportunities for teamwork and collaboration.

Because healthcare is complex, rapidly changing, and full of challenges, the historical fragmented approach to patient care delivery does not work in today's environment. Organizations that focus on creating cultures and structures to support interprofessional collaboration and opportunities to work together to improve design and workflow processes will have positive outcomes. Professional governance models that are inclusive to all professions support this vision.

The FLIGHT Model allows for the interprofessional team to share their unique understanding when a change is being explored. Professional Governance models that are only focused around nursing's perspectives are missing other key perspectives and may work on changes that are not reflective of the whole picture. Having an interprofessional approach can save time, energy, and costs. When you consider all disciplines and vantage points, you are more likely to implement a successful change and get it right the first time.

The Changing Face of Organizations

Today's workplace is in such a state of flux that almost everyone, no matter their industry, finds it hard to keep up. Competition has become fierce with an ever-increasing demand to lower labor and supply costs. If they have any hope of keeping up, organizations must be capable of changing direction quickly and appropriately to meet the demands of an increasingly fickle marketplace.

To complicate things further, organizations cannot take their workforce for granted. Today's employees are demanding more than pay and benefits; they want to be listened to, and they want to be involved in the decisions that affect them directly. They want work to be a fulfilling part of their lives, and they do not hesitate to change jobs to find that fulfillment.

Oddly enough, organizations that have been very successful in their fields often find it most difficult to change. Even though their historic success may have been built on a highly innovative idea, there is a common tendency to calcification: "We've been doing just fine with what we have; let's not mess with it" (Gryskiewicz, 1999). Table 1.1 compares organizational structure differences for the 20th and 21st centuries.

TABLE 1.1   A Comparison of Organizational Characteristics in the 20th and 21st Centuries

	Structure	Systems	Culture
20th-Century Organization	Bureaucratic Multi-leveled Organized with the expectation that senior management will manage Characterized by policies and procedures that create many complicated and internal interdependencies	Depend on few performance information systems Distribute performance data to executives only Offer management training and support systems to senior people only	Inwardly focused Centralized Slow to make decisions Political Risk averse
21st-Century Organization	Non bureaucratic, with fewer rules and employees Limited to fewer levels Organized with the expectation that management will lead, lower level employees will manage	Depend on many performance information systems, providing data on customers especially Distribute performance data widely Offer management training and support systems to many people	Externally oriented Empowering Quick to make decisions Open and candid More risk tolerant

(Adapted from Kotter, 2012)

Forces Affecting Healthcare Delivery

Some forces affecting healthcare delivery include:

- Multicultural and generational influences

- Changing patient demographics

- The changing face of healthcare finance

- The introduction of Lean and Six Sigma concepts into healthcare organizations

- The emerging understanding of the importance of the interprofessional team and high reliability techniques to ensure safe and effective communication between providers

In the following sections, we will touch briefly on each of the first three forces listed above, as they all play a part in why and how the FLIGHT Model is a relevant model for organizations today. The remaining two factors (the Lean and Six Sigma concepts, and the importance of the interprofessional team) will be explored in later chapters.

Multicultural and Generational Influences

We live in a diverse country. Organizations lucky enough to have a workforce as diverse as the population find themselves armed with many perspectives, views, and ideas that add strength to their ability to strategize, communicate, and perform improvement work. While it can be said that nurses are more similar than they are different, and despite the many common attributes that nurses share, there still exist cultural differences. For the purposes of this book, we define *culture* as a set of values, practices, traditions, or beliefs a group shares as learned through social interaction. Other factors that contribute to workplace diversity and cultural differences in the workplace are differences attributable to work styles.

There are a multitude of benefits that a multicultural workplace can bring to teams—and there are a couple of challenges as well. The benefits are spelled out in the next sections.

More Understanding and Respect for Cultural Differences

Employees learn to be more open-minded, flexible, and tolerant. Cultural differences discourage the use of "groupthink" as teams are exposed to new ideas and perspectives. Individuals get to see the world through other people's eyes. Cross-cultural understanding, along with local healthcare knowledge and understanding, allows for patient-centric (rather than individual-centric) solutions.

More Innovative and Creative Approaches to Problems and Problem-Solving

Teams that include members from multiple backgrounds and experiences work more creatively to innovate and solve problems (Abreu, 2014). The more your network includes individuals from different cultural backgrounds, the more you will be creatively stimulated by different ideas and perspectives. A variety of viewpoints, along with the wide-ranging personal and professional experience of an international team, can offer new perspectives that inspire colleagues to see the workplace—and the world—differently. Multiple voices, perspectives, and personalities bouncing off one another can give rise to out-of-the-box thinking. By offering a platform for the open exchange of ideas, organizations can reap the biggest benefits of diversity in the workplace. When people come together from different backgrounds and are encouraged to contribute ideas, innovation becomes the norm.

Better Service for Customers and Partners

A multicultural workforce can improve an organization's ability to connect and communicate with customers (patients and families). Employees who are part of a multicultural workforce generally are more sensitive to other cultures (Hamel, n.d.).

Diverse Teams Are More Productive and Perform Better

The range of experience, expertise, and working methods that a diverse workplace offers can boost problem-solving capacity and lead to greater productivity. In fact, studies have shown that organizations with a culture of diversity and inclusion are both happier and more productive (Brooks, 2011). When employees are happy and have reduced conflict, the path is cleared for more productivity and efficiency. Mutual respect and understanding create stronger teams and happier individuals who can focus on the job at hand, rather than getting mired down in feelings of harassment or suppression.

The Challenges of a Multicultural Workplace

Although the benefits to a multicultural workplace are significant, you cannot ignore the challenges. Some challenges include:

- Colleagues from some cultures may be less likely to let their voices be heard. This can be particularly challenging for colleagues from polite or deferential cultures who may feel less comfortable speaking up or sharing ideas, particularly if they are new to the team or in a more junior role. Conversely, assertive colleagues may be more inclined to speak up when others don't.

- Integration across multicultural teams can be difficult in the face of prejudice or negative cultural stereotypes. Negative cultural stereotypes can be seriously detrimental to an organization's or a team's morale and the ability to be productive. While outright prejudice or stereotyping is a serious concern, ingrained and unconscious cultural biases can be a more difficult challenge of workplace diversity to overcome. Even in a nondiverse workplace, exclusive social groups or cliques naturally happen; they happen more so in a diverse workforce. When such groups form, informal divisions can occur that will impede social integration. It can also lead to a situation where culturally diverse employees will avoid each other. This can hinder the effective sharing of knowledge, experience, and skills, resulting in decreased productivity, team efficacy, and productivity.

- Professional communication can be misinterpreted or difficult to understand across languages and cultures. There is a very real risk that communication can get lost in translation among multicultural colleagues. Language barriers are just one challenge. Even in an organization where everyone speaks English, comprehending a range of accents or understanding a native speaker's use of idioms can be difficult. Nonverbal communication is a delicate and nuanced part of cultural interaction that can lead to misunderstandings or even offense between team members from different cultures or countries. Things like comfortable levels of physical space, making or maintaining eye contact, and gesturing can all be vastly different across cultures.

- Conflicting working styles across teams can reduce productivity. Working styles and attitudes toward work can be very different, reflecting cultural values and compounding differences. Approaches to teamwork and collaboration can vary notably, with some cultures valuing collective consensus when working toward a goal and others emphasizing individual independence. Additionally, emphasis on order, rigor, and organization in the workplace versus flexibility and spontaneity can also reflect underlying cultural values.

• Challenges can also stem from employees' generational differences. A diverse workplace includes employees considered traditionalists, baby boomers, Generation X, and millennials. Each generation has distinct characteristics. In addition to the four generations listed here, a not-yet-named generation is emerging.

Based on the life experiences its members have shared, each generation has its own way of doing things and of viewing the world. These generational differences are evident in their perceptions of authority, views of leadership, workplace relationships, thoughts on loyalty, and even what "turns them off" (Clipper, 2013). Table 1.2 delineates generational differences.

TABLE 1.2 Generational Differences

	Size	Thoughts on Authority	Leadership Preference	Turnoffs	Loyalty to	Outlook	Relationships in the Workforce
Traditionalists	75 million	Respectful	Hierarchy	Vulgarity	Company or team	Practical	Don't have to like everyone
Boomers	80 million	Love/hate	Consensus	Politically incorrect	My need to succeed	Optimistic	Get along and fit in
Xers	46 million	Unimpressed	Competent	Hype, lies	People who help me with my career	Skeptical	Autonomous
Millennials	76 million	Polite	Pull team together	Promiscuity	My need for meaningful work	Hopeful	Seek mentors Large social network

(Clipper, 2013, p. 5)

The Aging Baby Boomer

Baby boomers are stimulating huge changes to the healthcare industry. Boomers make up roughly 75 million Americans, and approximately 3 million baby boomers will retire annually for the next 20 years. By 2029, the number of Americans 65 years or greater will grow to more than 71 million, a 73% overall increase from today (Barr, 2014). Inversely, baby boomers will leave the workforce in exponential numbers and transition from commercial healthcare plans to traditional Medicare retirement plans. The baby boomer generation has unique social and cultural values that will create tremendous challenges on how healthcare is delivered (Barr, 2014). Table 1.3 describes the impact of baby boomers on healthcare.

TABLE 1.3   The Impact of Baby Boomers on Healthcare in the US

Diversity	Baby boomers will require increased sensitivity to cultural differences as this population is more ethnically and racially diverse than past generations.
Education	Baby boomers seek more involvement with healthcare decision-making than previous generations and are very receptive to mobile healthcare options such as telemedicine and electronic visits.
Finances	Some baby boomers lost significant portions of financial savings during the great recession; thus, most boomers will make careful purchases as retirement age approaches.
Geography	Baby boomers will retire in popular states such as Arizona, California, Florida, North Carolina, and Texas, changing the healthcare profile of those locations.
Lifestyle	It is predicted that palliative care will grow as boomers will focus on activity and mobility as they age, with a new focus on complementary healthcare interventions.

(Barr, 2014)

Changing Patient Demographics

As nurses, we know that our patients and their families are increasingly more technologically savvy. When you walk into a hospital waiting area or into a hospital room, you often see patients and visitors looking down at their smartphones or on other mobile devices, using apps and web searches to find answers to health-related questions. It's estimated that 94% of consumers aged 18–29 use a smartphone, 89% of consumers aged 30–49 use a smartphone, 73% of consumers aged 50–64 use a smartphone, and 46% of adults over 65 use a smartphone (Pew Research Center, 2018). How often do you hear patients say, "I read this on the Internet," and "What do you think about this printout?" The increase in smartphone usage is changing how consumers utilize health-care services.

As healthcare providers, we are obligated to address this changing demographic. Dattilo et al. (2017) share that consumers enjoy using smartphones for health-related services such as appointment reminders, test results, communicating with members of the care team, and discharge instructions. One study suggested that 45% of consumers used their smartphone to find health-related information, 28% of consumers own some type of health app, yet only 11% of consumers are referred by a clinician to specific technological websites or apps (Dattilo et al., 2017).

Access to electronic health-related information is creating well-informed consumers. No longer are these consumers going with the grain. Patients often ask about recommendations and interventions before a healthcare provider has time to diagnose. And this consumer comes in ready with questions and thoughts. This information improves consumers' knowledge and often leads to more robust healthcare conversations.

While improved access to general health information and personal electronic health records is beneficial for patients and providers alike, there is a troublesome consumer demographic in healthcare facilities to consider—that of the disruptive patient. The disruptive patient poses unique challenges in providing optimal healthcare delivery. This demographic is closely associated with borderline personality symptomology, misuse of alcohol and/or drugs, and prescription medication misuse or abuse (Rosenstein, 2015). Healthcare consumers often experience stress, frustration, and emotionally charged events during hospitalizations, which increases the chance of aggressive or disruptive behavior (Van Den Bos, Creten, Davenport, & Roberts, 2017). Aggressive and disruptive behavior can lead to negative effects in healthcare, affect patient safety, and decrease employee satisfaction and morale (Petrovic & Scholl, 2018). From 2005 to 2014, the US Bureau of Labor Statistics reported that healthcare workplace violence increased by 110% (Advisory Board, 2016). This expanding demographic adds unique difficulties to caring for this population and should be considered when implementing change.

The Changing Landscape of Healthcare Finance

Today, no matter the industry, companies and organizations are realizing that the only way to see profitable growth is to cut costs, often dramatically. There is no safe harbor when it comes to the bottom line. As such, organizations are focusing on managing costs as rigorously as they concentrate on growing revenues. Welcome to the new normal. It doesn't matter if you are a for-profit or a not-for-profit organization; to be successful in today's environment, you must be fiscally sound.

Organizations that have a cost structure that is not aligned with the organization's strategy will base their spending on other factors—which may be a detriment to the organization. Additionally, if inefficiencies proliferate and the internal bureaucracy is so cumbersome that it takes a prolonged time to implement needed change or a new way of working, the competition may win the business. When decisions made weeks ago still have not been executed, information moves haltingly through the organization, people are afraid to take calculated risks for fear of failure and career derailment, and incentives don't motivate behaviors that drive the organization's strategic priorities, we all suffer (Couto, Plansky, & Caglar, 2017).

The FLIGHT Model has a cost associated with it. There is a defined budget that encourages unit-based leadership and change priorities. However, the cost of the FLIGHT Model should be considered a "good" cost (Couto et al., 2017). "The right way to think about costs is to align them with the strategic growth priorities of your business—those few capabilities that distinguish your (organization) and contribute disproportionately to its success. Those capabilities should be fully funded" (Couto et al., 2017, p. 19).

Adapting to Change

As the healthcare landscape changes, providers and institutions must find a way to change with it. The FLIGHT Model is a unit council structure that provides a framework within which practice changes and improvements can be implemented, with long-term sustainability. It's an inherently empowering model, encouraging change to originate from the frontline providers who know best the challenges they face and how to solve those challenges, in order to improve the work environment and provide optimal care to patients.

Nurses, in particular, are invaluable assets in leading change and inspiring others around them to do the same.

References

Abreu, K. (2014, December 9). The myriad benefits of diversity in the workplace. *Entrepreneur*. Retrieved from https://www.entrepreneur.com/article/240550

Advisory Board. (2016, December 7). *The alarming stats on violence against nurses*. Retrieved from https://www.advisory.com/daily-briefing/2016/12/07/violence-against-nurses

Barr, P. (2014, January 14). Baby boomers will transform health care as they age. *H&HN*. Retrieved from https://www.hhnmag.com/articles/5298-Boomers-Will-Transform-Health-Care-as-They-Age

Battié, R. N. (2013). The IOM report on the future of nursing: What perioperative nurses need to know. *AORN Journal, 98*(3), 227–234. doi: 10.1016/j.aorn.2013.07.007

Bridges, D. R., Davidson, R. A., Odegard, P. S., Maki, I. V., & Tomkowiak, J. (2011, April 8). Interprofessional collaboration: Three best practice models of interprofessional education. *Medical Education Online, 16*(1). doi: 10.3402/meo.v16i0.6035

Brooks, C. (2011, December 14). Diverse staffs are happier, more productive. *Business News Daily*. Retrieved from http://www.businessnewsdaily.com/1787-staff-hiring-diversity.html

Bureau of Labor Statistics, U.S. Department of Labor. (2015, July 13). Registered nurses have highest employment in healthcare occupations; anesthesiologists earn the most. *The Economics Daily*. Retrieved from https://www.bls.gov/opub/ted/2015/registered-nurses-have-highest-employment-in-healthcare-occupations-anesthesiologists-earn-the-most.htm

Clipper, B. (2013). *The nurse manager's guide to an intergenerational workforce*. Indianapolis, IN: Sigma Theta Tau International.

Committee on the Robert Wood Johnson Foundation Initiative on the Future of Nursing, Institute of Medicine. (2011). *Future of nursing: Leading change, advancing health* [ProQuest Ebook Central]. Retrieved from https://ebookcentral.proquest.com/lib/westerngovernorsebooks/reader.action?docID=3378745&ppg=1

Couto, V., Plansky, J., & Caglar, D. (2017). *Fit for growth: A guide to strategic cost cutting, restructuring, and renewal*. Hoboken, NJ: John Wiley & Sons, Inc.

Dattilo, J., Gittings, D., Sloan, M., Hardaker, W., Deasey, M., & Sheth, N. (2017). "Is there an app for that?" Orthopaedic patient preferences for a smartphone application. *Applied Clinical Informatics, 8*(3), 832–844. doi: 10.4338/ACI-2017-04-RA-0058

Dempsey, C., Reilly, B., & Buhlman, N. (2014). Improving the patient experience: Real-world strategies for engaging nurses. *The Journal of Nursing Administration, 44*(3), 142–151.

Gilbert, H. V., Yan, J., & Hoffman, S. J. (2010). A WHO report: Framework for action on interprofessional education and collaborative practice. *Journal of Allied Health, 39*(3), 196–197.

Gryskiewicz, S. S. (1999). *Positive turbulence: Developing climates for creativity, innovation, and renewal*. San Francisco, CA: Jossey-Bass.

Hamel, G. (n.d.). The advantages of a multicultural labor force. *Chron.com*. Retrieved from http://smallbusiness.chron.com/advantages-multicultural-labor-force-16678.html

Hovland, C. A., Whitford, M., & Niederriter, J. (2018). Interprofessional education: Insights from a cohort of nursing students. *Journal for Nurses in Professional Development, 31*(4), 219–225. doi: 10.1097/NND.0000000000000466

Ketelsen, L., Cook, K., & Kennedy, B. (2014). *The HCAHPS handbook: Tactics to improve quality and the patient experience.* Gulf Breeze, FL: Fire Starter Publishing.

Kotter, J. P. (2012). *Leading change.* Boston, MA: *Harvard Business Review.*

Medicare Learning Network, CMS.gov. (2017). *Hospital value-based purchasing.* Retrieved from https://www.cms.gov/Outreach-and-Education/Medicare-Learning-Network-MLN/MLNProducts/downloads/Hospital_VBPurchasing_Fact_Sheet_ICN907664.pdf

Nickitas, D. M., Middaugh, D. J., & Aries, N. (Eds.). (2016). *Policy and politics for nurses and other health professionals: Advocacy and action.* Sudbury, MA: Jones & Bartlett.

O'Rourke, M. W. (2003). Rebuilding a professional practice model: The return of role-based practice accountability. *Nursing Administrative Quarterly, 27*(2), 95–105.

Petrovic, M. A., & Scholl, A. T. (2018). Why we need a single definition of disruptive behavior. *Cureus, 10*(3), e2339. doi: 10.7759/cureus.2339

Pew Research Center. (2018, February 5). *Mobile fact sheet.* Retrieved from http://www.pewinternet.org/fact-sheet/mobile/

Rosenstein, A. H. (2015). Addressing the causes and consequences of disruptive behaviors in the healthcare setting. *Journal of Psychology & Clinical Psychiatry, 3*(3). doi: 10.15406/jpcpy.2015.03.00136

Siwicki, B. (2017, December 19). Biggest EHR challenges for 2018: Security, interoperability, clinician burnout. *Healthcare IT News.* Retrieved from https://www.healthcareitnews.com/news/biggest-ehr-challenges-2018-security-interoperability-clinician-burnout

Van Den Bos, J., Creten, N., Davenport, S., & Roberts, M. (2017, July 26). Cost of community violence to hospitals and health systems. *American Hospital Association.* Retrieved from https://www.aha.org/guidesreports/2018-01-18-cost-community-violence-hospitals-and-health-systems

World Health Organization. (2010). *Framework for action on interprofessional education and collaborative practice.* Retrieved from https://apps.who.int/iris/bitstream/handle/10665/70185/WHO_HRH_HPN_10.3_eng.pdf?sequence=1

"The leader is one who mobilizes others toward a goal shared by leaders and followers... Leaders, followers and goals make up the three equally necessary supports for leadership."

–Gary Wills

2

THE EVOLUTION OF GOVERNANCE MODELS

History of Shared Governance

The shared governance model was introduced in the early 1980s and is a continually evolving framework that supports professional nursing practice and decision-making. Within a shared governance structure, clinical nurses experience autonomy and are empowered and supported by organizational leadership to tackle issues that affect their practice. A successfully designed governance structure can lead to improved clinical outcomes, improved employee satisfaction and retention rates, future leadership development, and increased employee engagement (Caramanica, 2004; Porter O'Grady & Finnigan, 1984; Porter O'Grady & Malloch, 2003; Porter O'Grady & Wilson, 1995).

Professional governance is as much a structure and a process as it is an ideology. For professional governance to be fully functional, a structural foundation is required to allow and encourage ideas and work to flow without unnecessary barriers. Ideally, this structure includes decision-making at the bedside, through unit councils, as well as decision-making at the organization level, through hospital-wide councils. The intention of professional governance at the unit level is to give every clinical nurse the opportunity to be involved in their practice and to have a clear path to champion an idea for change. Professional governance is the structure that allows the thoughts, perspectives, expertise, and influence of clinical nurses to be at the table regarding decisions around nursing practice and the practice environment. Professional governance, when compared to traditional governance, allows for decisions and influence to be closer to the point of care and encourages teamwork, partnerships, and a spirit of engagement. See Table 2.1 for a comparison of the two.

TABLE 2.1   Professional Governance Compared to Traditional Governance

Traditional Governance	Professional Governance
Position-based	Knowledge-based
Distant from point of care/service	Occurs at point of care/service
Hierarchical communication	Direct communication
Limited employee input	High employee input
Separates responsibility/managers are accountable	Integrates equity, accountability, and authority for employees and managers
Us-them work environment	Synergistic work environment

Divided goals/purpose	Cohesive goals/purpose, ownership
Independent activities/tasks	Collegiality, collaboration, partnership

(HCPro, 2007)

Professional Governance Concepts

The specific way an organization structures governance can vary and yet be quite successful. While there is no ideal structure, a successful structure creates an environment where nurses and interprofessional partners *want* to practice. According to Porter O'Grady, Hawkins, and Parker (1997), when an organization embraces professional governance concepts, the culture shifts toward work that supports the following principles:

- Partnership

- Equity

- Accountability

- Ownership

Partnership

The principle of *partnership* centers on building relationships between stakeholders and ensuring all key players are present and at the table when discussing change. The perspectives of nursing leaders, clinical nurses, interprofessional partners, and patients and family members are valued when considering solutions to issues. These strong partnerships ensure that issues are evaluated from multiple perspectives and that the final decision has the optimal opportunity for success. When healthy partnerships exist, outcomes are better, and processes are stronger.

A Note on Terminology

Change is continual and ongoing. When we started our journey with the FLIGHT Model, the terminology used was *shared governance*. A shift toward *professional governance* is taking place in the literature. We embrace this changing terminology and believe it supports our vision of professional nurses working with interprofessional teams. In most instances in this book, you will find we use *professional governance* with the exception of direct quotes or situations where a historical perspective is better served with *shared governance*.

FLIGHT Simulator: Partnership in Action

Time is extremely valuable when caring for a patient with an ST-Elevation Myocardial Infarction (STEMI). Good communication and smooth transitions are essential to provide the patient with the life-saving intervention he needs. Cath Lab employees partnered with Emergency Department employees to improve the process of transitioning a STEMI patient from the Emergency Department (ED) to the Cardiac Cath Lab. During this work, they defined roles and re-sponsibilities and necessary communication. After reviewing several options, the project team decided to add a whiteboard in the Cath Lab for the ED RN to record relevant patient information while the patient is getting prepared for his procedure. This simple change saved valuable time and improved communication. Input from both departments and all disciplines involved in caring for a STEMI pa-tient was necessary for the success of this work.

Equity

The principle of *equity* is based on the belief that every role is important, and no one role or perspective holds more influence than another. The focus moves from power gradients driving decisions to decision-making around the point of care with the focus on improving structures and processes. Equity enhances partnerships and ultimately improves the work environment and clinical out-comes.

FLIGHT Simulator: Equity in Action

Interprofessional communication surrounding the plan of care is essential. Every day in the critical care and step-down units, a team of physicians, nurses, and other interprofessional partners round on their patients and discuss the plan of care. Although everyone has a different role and knowledge base, the power gradient is level and one perspective does not dominate over the others. Respect of other roles and perspectives as well as clear, professional commu-nication that centers around doing the right thing for the patient is the focus of the rounding.

Accountability

The principle of *accountability* is core to the success of a governance model. In traditional governance, decisions about change and how to implement it are typically directed by leaders to their employees. Often the result is frustration—frustration by employees who may see a better way and frustration by leaders when expected results are not achieved. Within professional governance, clinical nurses are empowered to make decisions that affect care delivery, quality and safety, professional practice, and their work environment. With role clarity and a focus on outcomes and partnerships, accountability is shared, and individuals involved in the change feel valued and appreciated for their contributions.

FLIGHT Simulator: Accountability in Action

Nurses know that hourly rounding is best for their patients and can decrease call light volumes, reduce falls, and improve patient satisfaction (Halm, 2009). One medical/surgical unit knew the upside of hourly rounding but had a hard time holding people accountable to consistently round on their own patients. The current setup made it hard to be successful. One RN witnessed another hospital organize its hourly rounding differently; the unit signed up for time slots and rounded on half of the unit. This RN thought, "We could do this here!" and created a plan, gained input from her peers, and implemented a new approach. Adjustments were made throughout the implementation period based on realities and feedback. Leadership supported her throughout the process, helped remove barriers, and celebrated the successes with the unit employees.

Ownership

Ownership is the personal commitment made to support the vision and the work of the organization. There is an acceptance of the importance of everyone's work and the understanding that an organization's success depends on the ability and evidence of individual employees to perform at the highest level of competence and skill.

FLIGHT Simulator: Ownership in Action

Reduction of hospital-acquired infections is a universal focus. In one hospital, monitoring of hand hygiene compliance demonstrated inconsistent performance by all members of the healthcare team. Despite mantras of "gel in, gel out" and "wash your hands, save a life," the consistent personal commitment by all team members was lacking. The organization launched a Hand Hygiene campaign to highlight and educate all team members, including patients and family members, on their individual role and responsibility in ensuring proper hand hygiene for the protection of all. Leveling the playing field ensured that no individual was exempt from this practice. The message went out that everyone had a personal responsibility to remind others about proper hand hygiene no matter their role on the team or the perceived hierarchy. Educating the team and the patients/families about the importance of hand hygiene promoted ownership of the task. This increase in ownership resulted in improved hand hygiene compliance, which contributed to an overall reduction in hospital-acquired infections.

Current Influences Affecting Shared Governance

Shared governance has evolved through the years and has been influenced by various theoretical perspectives. Organizational, leadership, management, and even sociological theories have all influenced the concepts and appearance of shared governance today (Anthony, 2004). How each organization opts to create and support their governance structure is individualized. In the early phases of implementing governance, the structure is often customized to fit the organizational priorities and culture, typically building both hospital-wide councils and unit councils. The membership, makeup, and scope of each council can vary greatly depending on the needs of the organization. As shared governance matures through the years, it is common for the council structure to transform based on feedback and to meet the changing needs of the organization. Because of this variability and fluidity, there is a wide range of approaches to a council structure and a wide range of successes and failures (Anthony, 2004; Caramanica, 2004). One consistent theme, however, is that the professional nurse's engagement and buy-in are key to creating an empowered organization and ensuring professional governance success.

Challenges With the Traditional Model

When an organization decides to implement shared governance, it often wants to increase nurse participation in changes to care delivery and the work environment. The organization's governance pioneers seek out information on best practices and explore how other organizations have built their structures. The traditional model typically is implemented. Both hospital-wide councils and unit councils are created, and members are recruited and commit to being on the council for a set amount of time. Routine meetings (usually monthly) are scheduled, and there is a hope that the council can produce change.

The traditional model can work, and there are numerous articles on how to be most effective. Organizations with abundant resources, engaged clinical nurses, and leadership support can be set for success. The current reality, however, is that organizations are looking at many ways to reduce costs while rapidly driving change and keeping employees engaged. Healthcare has dramatically changed in the last 20 years, and the traditional governance model has not. Innovative adjustments to the traditional model are necessary to meet current demands of the healthcare environment (French-Bravo & Crow, 2015).

In addition to the rapidly changing healthcare environment, the generational mix of clinical nurses is expanding, and new ways of thinking are being introduced. Generation X and the millennials are seeking work-life balance and want to have flexibility in their commitments (Clipper, 2013). These generations see opportunity for nontraditional approaches to getting work done and do not necessarily see meetings as an effective use of their time. Furthermore, committing to a one- or two-year term on a council can be challenging. Many clinical nurses want to be involved with governance and changes they believe in but are uncertain about how much time it will take and whether their personal life will allow them to be involved in a meaningful way. The interested nurse may have experience in seeing council members take work home without being paid—which is a deterrent. These situations can limit the engagement of highly motivated and talented clinical nurses.

The cost of shared governance can be a concern for many organizations. Leaders want to see a return on their investment with productive work that is aligned with the strategic plan and current initiatives. For this to occur, leaders need to understand how to support shared governance, and council members need to have a clear understanding of what their role is and have knowledge about how to develop and implement a plan for change and how to evaluate its effectiveness. When there is a lack of knowledge, unclear focus, and scattered leadership support, shared governance is very costly and difficult to sustain.

There is no simple recipe for success with implementing and supporting a professional governance structure, but essential components need to be in place to create a culture where ideas truly flow from the bedside and employees are engaged and committed to their role, their team, and the patients and families they serve. The following chapters will describe a new approach to unit-based professional governance. The FLIGHT Model was created to meet the changing demands and current realities of the healthcare environment, to address the concerns of a diverse workforce, and to acknowledge the importance of working as an interprofessional team when creating change. Organizations need their employees to be engaged and to be a part of the transformation in optimizing the delivery of care and the work environments. The FLIGHT Model is one approach to do this important work.

Evaluating Established Governance Models: What Needs to Change?

Many healthcare organizations have adopted a traditional governance model that includes both unit councils and councils that represent the entire organization. This traditional model has often been in place for many years with little or no revisions. We have observed that often hospital or organization-wide councils seemed to flourish while unit councils were fraught with frustration and burnout from both council and noncouncil members.

Is your organization experiencing any of these common issues?

- Unit council chairs feeling pressure to show results yet council members largely deferring to the chair for most of the work.
- Projects are created because of employee complaints, yet no solutions are brought forward.
- Projects often take months, if not years, to complete.
- Attendance at unit council meetings is sporadic at best.
- Members are not volunteering for a project or work outside of the council meeting time.

- Council members are not given dedicated time to work on projects—leading to members feeling unsupported and unwilling to give more.

- Clinical nurses find it difficult to commit to the membership term (typically two years).

- Council members often half-heartedly stay beyond their two-year term due to failed recruitment efforts.

- Nurses on the council are often viewed as a "clique" by those outside the council.

- Unit council projects are often not aligned with organizational goals.

Synergistic Work Environment

A synergistic work environment is a key differentiator in organizations that embrace professional governance. Synergy is teamwork, open-mindedness, and the adventure of finding new solutions to old problems. In the FLIGHT Model, team members can share their personal experiences and expertise. Rather than a finite number of minds contributing, the field is widened to include an entire team. Harris, Roussel, Thomas, and Dearman (2016) discuss a synergistic work environment:

> While difficult to define, synergy is a product of effective work teams. Such an experience is commonly cited as one of the benefits and satisfiers realized when working in a highly effective team. As individuals become members of a team and successfully work through the developmental stages, their energy, respect, and anticipation of positive outcomes buoy the members as they recognize the products and outcomes of coming together. Additionally, the enthusiasm and spirit of possibility are shared with individuals outside the work team while sharing experiences and implementing change. (pp. 87–88)

In a synergistic environment, multiple disciplines come together to produce something greater than what one could achieve on one's own. Engagement by a whole team allows for richer conversations, wiser decisions, and more rapid results. Synergy allows the opportunity to create new understandings that one may be less likely to discover in solitude.

A highly functioning unit council structure empowers employees and allows for creative cooperation in an energizing way. When you encourage employees to create the ideas, and then you listen to their ideas and allow them to work in a flexible manner to produce results, the overall outcomes are beneficial to all. Implementing the FLIGHT Model requires a synergistic environment in which all members are encouraged to participate. Including disciplines that may have previously been excluded in the traditional unit council provides exponentially greater success to any project. Interprofessional collaboration can lead to improved patient outcomes and quality of care; this kind of collaboration is characteristic of highly successful healthcare innovation (Stephen, 2015). It is important to realize the benefits associated with encouraging and providing an inclusive environment. A synergistic environment yields greater innovative ideas, ultimately leading to greater transformational change. Erickson, Jones, and Ditomassi (2013) describe innovation with four key assumptions:

> Innovation and entrepreneurial teamwork are critical to the creation of a professional environment that embraces change. As healthcare clinicians, we need to innovate and make certain that the delivery of patient care and structures that support it change to meet the changing populations we serve. Regarding innovation, several key assumptions are stated:
>
> - Innovation takes great leaders.
> - Imagination is necessary and fun for innovation to occur.
> - Collaborative decision-making is a core value.
> - Patient-centered care is key. (p. 31)

Healthcare organizations are being asked to increase productivity and improve patient and quality outcomes and efficiency, all while reducing costs. Change is inevitable and necessary, especially in today's environment. Some people adapt well to change and welcome its process; others will avoid it and look for failures along the way. How does an organization with diverse employees with varied backgrounds and experiences use change to positively transform? We believe the FLIGHT Model of unit-based professional governance can be instrumental in supporting a culture change and in providing clinical nurses a chance to participate and lead transformational change.

The FLIGHT Model: A New Approach to Professional Governance

The FLIGHT Model is a type of professional governance model, with some important innovations to address the challenges of today's healthcare environment. FLIGHT stands for Fostering Leadership, Innovation, and Growth through Healthcare Teams. The FLIGHT Model empowers the clinical nurse to turn creative solutions into action. With this model, nurses are engaged and involved in important decisions related to clinical outcomes, their work environment, and workflow. The FLIGHT Model is predicated on the notion that all members of the healthcare team have a role and a responsibility to improve patient care outcomes and the work environment, including their own work satisfaction. This work should not be left to a defined group of individuals who compose a traditional unit council—it should be shared across the department. Additionally, the FLIGHT Model encourages creativity and expression of individual passion by allowing interprofessional team members to be owners of projects that are important to them and that are within the scope of their expertise. This inclusive model is a response to the individuality that each team member brings to the work setting, to patient care, and to the cohesiveness of the team.

Innovative ideas and process changes should ideally germinate from clinical employees because those clinicians and employees closest to the patient and to the workflow know the realities and daily challenges of their work. They are in the unique position of clearly seeing what is working and what is broken and are best able to explore innovative approaches as colleagues. When a healthcare organization is not structured to allow ideas to flow from the bedside, clinical employees are left feeling disempowered and only as the recipients of change—not the drivers of change.

The FLIGHT Model supports and develops leaders and leadership skills, which promotes professional development. Leading change at any level provides the opportunity to gain insight into and expertise with project management, group dynamics, organizational politics, and other leadership skills. The model also supports projects of any size. Often employees begin their journeys by completing a small unit council project with success. Success at a small level can lead to increased confidence and willingness to tackle a larger-scale project. With every project, employees experience the project workflow, hone their leadership skills, and learn the intricacies of leading through change. The FLIGHT Model provides employees with leadership skills that enable them to develop professionally and advance their careers when they are ready. Many project leads have been subsequently promoted to advanced positions, and many unit council chairs have accepted formal leadership positions on their units.

The FLIGHT Model supports the selection of unit-based projects that are in alignment with organizational goals. When this occurs, all parties benefit. Patients and families benefit by improved care processes that are embraced successfully by clinical employees and that lead to improved outcomes. Employees benefit when changes advance or enhance workflow processes. The organization benefits with improved patient outcomes and cost-saving measures supported by employees.

In the next chapter, we take an in-depth look at the FLIGHT Model.

References

Anthony, M. K. (January 31, 2004). Shared governance models: The theory, practice, and evidence. *Online Journal of Issues in Nursing, 9*(1), Manuscript 4.

Caramanica, L. (January 31, 2004). Shared governance: Hartford Hospital's experience. *Online Journal of Issues in Nursing, 9*(1), Manuscript 2. Retrieved from http://ojin. nursingworld.org/MainMenuCategories/ANAMarketplace/ANAPeriodicals/OJIN/Tableof-Contents/Volume92004/No1Jan04/HartfordHospitalsExperience.html

Clipper, B. (2013). *The nurse manager's guide to an inter-generational workforce.* Indianapolis, IN: Sigma Theta Tau International.

Erickson, J. I., Jones, D. A., & Ditomassi, M. (2013). *Fostering nurse-led care: Professional practice for the bedside leader from Massachusetts General Hospital.* Indianapolis, IN: Sigma Theta Tau International.

French-Bravo, M., & Crow, G. (2015, March 19). Shared governance: The role of buy-in in bringing about change. *OJIN: The Online Journal of Issues in Nursing, 20*(2), 8. doi: 10.3912/OJIN.Vol20No02PPT02

Halm, M. A. (2009). Hourly rounds: What does the evidence indicate? *American Journal of Critical Care, 18*(6), 581–584. doi: 10.4037/ajcc2009350

Harris, J. L., Roussel, L., Thomas, P. L., & Dearman, C. (2016). *Project planning and management: A guide for nurses and interprofessional teams* (2nd ed.). Burlington, MA: Jones & Bartlett Learning.

HCPro, Inc. (2007, September 24). *Shared governance in practice: Strategies to build a staff-driven model of decision and action.* Retrieved from audioconference.

Porter-O'Grady, T., & Finnigan, S. (1984). *Shared governance for nursing: A creative approach to accountability.* Rockville, MD: Aspen Publishers.

Porter-O'Grady, T., Hawkins, M. A., & Parker, M. L. (Eds.). (1997). *Whole-systems shared governance: Architecture for integration.* Gaithersburg, MD: Aspen Publishers.

Porter-O'Grady, T., & Malloch, K. (2003). *Quantum leadership: A textbook of new leadership*. Sudbury, MA: Jones & Bartlett.

Porter-O'Grady, T., & Wilson, C. (1995). *The leadership revolution in health care: Altering systems, changing behaviors*. Gaithersburg, MD: Aspen Publishers.

Stephen, A. (2015, August 8). Fostering interprofessional collaboration in health care. *Campaign for Action*. Retrieved from https://campaignforaction.org/fostering-interprofessional-collaboration-healthcare/

2

MASTERING AERODYNAMICS

3

THE FLIGHT MODEL: AN IN-DEPTH LOOK

OBJECTIVES

- Understand underlying concepts of model success
- Differentiate between traditional-model project flow and new-model project flow
- Identify key components of the model
- Identify key roles and responsibilities

Parallels are often drawn between the aviation and healthcare industries due to their high-risk, high-tech natures; both require precise knowledge and skill, while at the same time having a certain dependence on instinct and intuition. Both industries are responsible for the safety of large numbers of people, and both can cause catastrophic events should something go wrong. Both require complete and specific communication among a wide array of professionals and support employees.

As stated in Chapter 2, FLIGHT stands for Fostering Leadership, Innovation, and Growth through Healthcare Teams. The FLIGHT Model image (see Figure 3.1) was developed to illustrate a unit council structure in which members of an interprofessional team must work closely together to ensure that an idea for change takes flight and stays on course for long-lasting improvement.

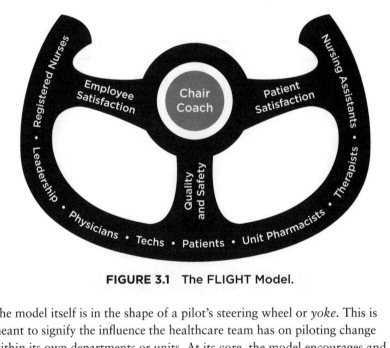

FIGURE 3.1   The FLIGHT Model.

The model itself is in the shape of a pilot's steering wheel or *yoke*. This is meant to signify the influence the healthcare team has on piloting change within its own departments or units. At its core, the model encourages and promotes the concept that any one individual, with a great idea, can and should be the pilot of change.

In the FLIGHT Model, all members of the healthcare team have a role and a responsibility to work together to lead a change. All interprofessional partners are part of the unit council and could potentially be project leads or project team members. This inclusive aspect is represented by the outer circle of the yoke.

The spokes of the pilot yoke indicate how organizational alignment is evidenced. All accepted/approved projects are categorized as either a project that will improve outcomes related to quality, improve the patient experience or patient satisfaction, or improve the work environment or employee satisfaction. Organizational alignment helps to ensure necessary resources to complete projects are not in opposition to competing priorities for the organization and helps to ensure barriers will be removed and successful completion of a project is optimized.

The unit council chair and coach are at the center of the yoke. The chair is a clinical nurse who works at the bedside and with all members of the interprofessional team. The coach is a charge nurse on the unit who provides leadership and coaching to ensure the chair has the support needed for successful project management. The use of registered nurses in the chair and coach role is deliberate. Registered nurses are educated and experienced in managing the care of patients within an interprofessional environment. They understand the importance each discipline brings to the department/unit and can uniquely support improvement efforts by all team members.

What Makes the FLIGHT Model Innovative?

The FLIGHT Model is designed to be deployed within acute care medical facilities at the unit or department level. However, it would have applicability in outpatient, ambulatory, behavioral health, and even home health or hospice settings. It is a model born out of a need to have an inclusive and broad engagement in professional governance by those who are closest to our patients. It, at its most fundamental, encourages participation and inclusion in decisions that affect patient care, the work environment, and the workflow of all team members who participate in the care of patients. The FLIGHT Model differs from a traditional unit council governance model in some important ways:

- The traditional, formal unit council with a defined membership has been abolished in the FLIGHT Model. All interprofessional members of a unit or department compose the unit council. With the abolishment of a defined unit council membership, it is no longer necessary to have formal unit council meetings. The costs associated with a formal unit council meeting have been shifted to costs surrounding project leads and project members.

- All members of the interprofessional care team that care for a patient population on a unit or department are considered part of the unit council. Literally, everyone who interacts with patients for a specific unit is now a member of that unit's council and can bring forth and lead projects that influence patient satisfaction, patient outcomes, and employee satisfaction.

- Any member of the healthcare team can become a project lead. A project lead spearheads a specific project and works within the FLIGHT Model to ensure organizational alignment, to implement within an agreed-upon time frame, and to maintain project costs within budget. The project lead works directly and closely with the council chair and coach to ensure success.

- Alignment with organizational goals and initiatives is a foundational construct within the FLIGHT Model, and all projects are evaluated to ensure alignment.

- Although there remains a council chair and a council coach, these individuals function like project managers. They work with the project leads to ensure successful completion of projects within a defined time frame and within a defined budget. The chair and coach have moved from being successful at running meetings in the traditional model to being successful at managing multiple projects in the FLIGHT Model.

- Budgeted dollars for work in the FLIGHT Model have shifted. Most of the budgeted dollars in the traditional unit council structure were used for nonproductive hours spent on council members attending monthly council meetings. In the FLIGHT Model, budgeted dollars are spent to allow project leads and project team members dedicated time to develop and implement a project. Unit council chairs are also provided dedicated time to work with each project lead to ensure successful implementation of projects. The overall budget for professional governance does not change—just how those dollars are used.

- In the FLIGHT Model, accountability for improvement efforts lies within the entire unit and not within the group of a finite membership of a traditional unit council. Ideas for change or improvement are generated by individuals who "own" the process. Any interprofessional member of the unit can identify a need for change or improvement. Once identified, the professional is expected to complete an intake tool fashioned after the Situation/Background/Assessment/Recommendation (SBAR) reporting tool. (See Chapter 7 and Appendix B for more detailed information regarding the SBAR tool.) The SBAR helps direct individuals to think globally and to use available resources and best practice evidence to support the need for change. Individuals can no longer "dump" a problem on a unit council and expect others to "fix" their issues. Accountability now rests with the entire team to "fix" quality and other issues.

The Four Pillars of the FLIGHT Model

Through the creation of our new unit council, we identified four pillars of the FLIGHT Model. These are:

- Engagement of interprofessional employees
- Supportive leadership
- Effective communication
- Alignment with organizational goals

These are the ingredients or the "secret sauce" we believe to be essential for implementation and sustainment of an improved, successful unit council structure. Figure 3.2 is a visual depiction of these pillars with "readiness for change" as the foundation. Keep these pillars in mind when evaluating your own organization's or unit's readiness for change (see Chapter 5).

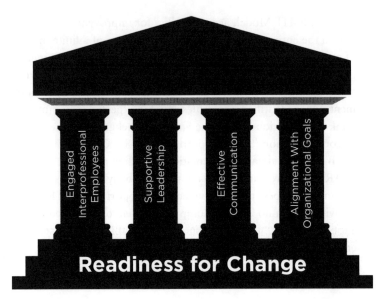

FIGURE 3.2   The four pillars of the FLIGHT Model.

Engaged Interprofessional Employees

When employees are involved with, committed to, and passionate about their work, they experience high levels of work engagement (Attridge, 2009). This engagement can be improved by adopting certain characteristics that support employees. In turn, an engaged workforce is beneficial for the entire organization, not just the employee. A culture that promotes teamwork, considerate treatment of employees, professional growth opportunities, flexible working practices, and good leadership and management practices fosters employee engagement (Devi, 2009).

Projects do not succeed if employees are not engaged. Ensuring your employees feel valued, respected, and encouraged to share their thoughts in a constructive way creates an environment that allows for free exchanges and robust dialogue. A healthy and positive working environment allows for employees to be part of the conversation. The success of the FLIGHT Model is predicated on engaged employees who want to be involved, who want to make a difference, and who are passionate about their work. Promoting the unit council membership as inclusive of all employees allows for an increase in potential solutions. When employees are engaged in their work, it encourages brainstorming and generation of more ideas for change, both in numbers of proposals as well as in numbers of projects that go to development. When employees are the drivers of change, they feel more ownership of the outcome and professional fulfillment by being connected and making a difference.

Supportive Leadership

In his book about teamwork, John Maxwell states, "The single biggest way to impact an organization is to focus on leadership development. There is almost no limit to the potential of an organization that recruits good people, raises them up as leaders and continually develops them" (Maxwell, 2001, p. 185). A clinical employee will not be successful without the support of leadership. A supportive leadership team is one that encourages and promotes increased employee engagement and empowerment. Whether the project is small or big, the process of change requires someone in a formal leadership position to be supportive and aid in the transformation.

> ### FLIGHT Team Check-In
>
> Many employees have creative solutions to specific problems they see every day, but how do you support them in sharing their ideas for change? As a clinical employee, do you feel supported in your work environment? As a leader, what can you do to increase engagement among employees?

Through the implementation of the FLIGHT Model, the clinical nurse who proposed an idea for a new unit council structure met with different levels of the nursing leadership team to share her thoughts. Because she garnered the support of key leaders, she was able to advance her idea, and a team was created to guide the change.

While the idea for a project may be born from an employee complaint, the FLIGHT Model's process provides the employee an opportunity to communicate both the complaint and a possible solution. That communication and dialogue spur the beginning of a chain of events leading to change. If the employee is unable to provide a recommendation to address the complaint, the FLIGHT Model expects engagement with the interprofessional team to brainstorm a possible solution—one that meets organizational goals and regulatory standards. A supportive leader can guide employees in this process, thereby provide mentoring and professional growth.

> ### FLIGHT Team Check-In
>
> Are you a leader that employees feel they can come to with an idea? Are you an employee that feels supported by your leadership team?

Effective Communication

Proper communication allows for a transfer of information and honesty and is vital for building a culture of transparency between management and employees. Strengthening communication can engage employees in the organization's priorities (Mishra, Boynton, & Mishra, 2014). Employees want to know the why's and how's behind leadership solutions. At the same time, employers should know the positives as well as the challenges happening in their work environment. Three benefits of strengthening communication include: employee motivation, collaboration and teamwork, and increased problem resolution. It is important to foster an environment that encourages employees to voice their opinions and believe that what they have to say matters. This will create a stronger and more positive working environment (Mattson, 2017).

Effective communication allows for increased employee motivation. It is important to know what drives individual employees because this directly affects their work. When communication is clear, employees know what is expected, can identify the common goal, and feel as though they have something to work toward. Lastly, effective communication enhances problem resolution and allows employees an opportunity to identify an issue before it turns into something larger (Mattson, 2017). Establishing a culture of communication is necessary to create a positive work environment—one that will flourish when every individual is on the same page.

> **FLIGHT Team Check-In**
>
> How is information disseminated in your organization? How can you improve this process, so employees feel involved? Are you a leader who communicates effectively to your team? Are you an employee member who is open to communication, and do you feel you receive adequate and up-to-date information that is necessary for your job?

Alignment With Organizational Goals

Strategic alignment in an organization can help ensure that resources are allocated correctly. Projects are less likely to be undertaken if they aren't aligned with the long-term vision of the organization, and this alignment can be useful as a recruiting tool because the organization can promise the mobile workforce the opportunity to work on much more high-value projects.

–Dave Wakeman (2015, para. 3)

In redesigning your unit council, it is important to align your projects with organizational goals. Collecting empirical data is imperative in determining the success of the project. Data can be garnered from employee surveys, patient outcomes, patient surveys, or other sources. In our previous unit council structure, we realized that many of our unit council projects stemmed from employee complaints, and the projects were not closely aligned with our organizational priorities. Once we aligned our project areas with the overarching organizational goals, employees were able to connect the dots between the impact of their projects and the bigger picture. When employees can clearly identify how their work aligns with the goals of the organization, they begin to feel part of something bigger—which promotes further engagement.

When we share organizational goals with employees and educate them about outcomes and data, ideas for improvement and projects begin to flourish. A supportive leader understands the importance of this and engages with the employees to incorporate organizational priorities into daily focus. This engages everyone to focus on a common vision and supports positive growth. Through proper organizational alignment, projects become more meaningful, and engaged employees feel a sense of purpose and accomplishment.

> ### FLIGHT Team Check-In
>
> As a leader, are your projects aligned with your organizational strategy? As an employee, do you know what your organizational goals are? Do your unit council projects fall under these categories?

The FLIGHT Model is predicated on the notion that all members of the healthcare team have a role and a responsibility to improve patient care outcomes, improve the work environment including their own work satisfaction, as well as improve the patient experience for those who are cared for on their unit. This work should not be left to a defined group of individuals who compose a traditional unit council—it should be shared across the department. Additionally, the FLIGHT Model encourages creativity and expression of individual passion by allowing interprofessional team members to be owners of projects that are important to them and that are within the scope of their expertise. This inclusive model literally is a response to the individuality that each team member brings to the work setting, to patient care, and to the cohesiveness of the team. The FLIGHT Model is designed to empower and engage employees across departments.

The FLIGHT Model in Action: Project Flow

Project flow and communication look very different between a traditional unit-based council and the FLIGHT Model of unit council professional governance. Although any member of a unit could identify a problem, in the traditional unit council structure, those problems are then presented to an identified group of nurses who compose the unit council. It is often expected that the unit council would "fix" the problem. Often there is no expectation that solutions be brought to the council as well as the problem. Multiple ideas or problems are presented, and the council then votes, or chooses in some manner, what projects to work on. Once chosen, the council members are expected to develop, implement, and evaluate project work as a council; they rarely enlist those outside the unit council. Figure 3.3 illustrates this flow visually.

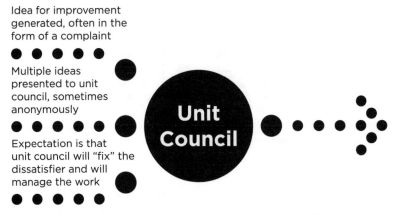

FIGURE 3.3   Traditional unit council project flow.

In the FLIGHT Model of unit-based professional governance, the flow is quite different. Any member of the team can identify a problem or a project and propose that project to the chair/coach of the unit council. By completing an SBAR, both the problem and at least one possible solution are defined. The person who presents the SBAR is often recruited to be the team lead, and projects are chosen based on alignment with organizational goals and budgetary allowances. Project flow is not linear, but rather inclusive and circular. Figure 3.4 illustrates this flow visually.

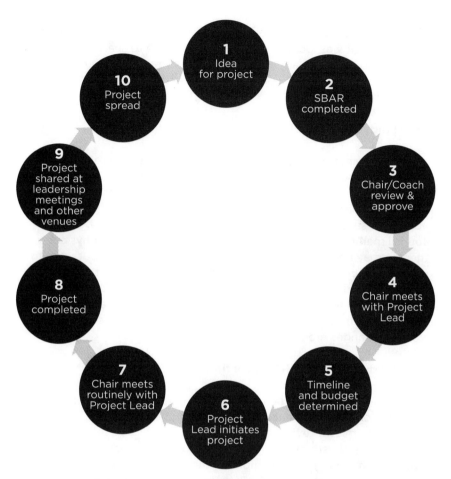

FIGURE 3.4   The FLIGHT Model project flow.

CASE STUDY: Comparing Traditional Unit Council Versus the FLIGHT Model in Practice

To illustrate how this looks in practice, let's examine two case studies—both dealing with the same issue.

John, an RN on a busy postoperative orthopedic unit, has just been to a conference and learned about a fall prevention intervention that he feels would benefit the patients on his unit. The intervention involves standardizing the placement of the gait belt in every patient's room.

This would allow all disciplines working with the patient to know where the belt was located. They would not have to search for gait belts, would not bring additional gait belts into the patient room, and would hopefully be more compliant with using the gait belt when ambulating patients.

Case Study A: The traditional unit council flow

John determines who the members of the unit council are and shares his idea with Ann, one of the members of the council. Ann promises John they will discuss the idea at the next unit council meeting. The unit council had just met, so it was three weeks later that Ann was able to present John's idea for standardization of the gait belts. The council members, not having all the information, felt that physical therapy may be in opposition to the intervention and did not want to pursue further. After the meeting, Ann advises John that the project has been discussed and the council was not in support. John was frustrated and felt as if his idea was not given sufficient attention. He thought to himself, "This is the last time I'm going to present an idea. Nothing changes around here."

Case Study B: The FLIGHT Model flow

John tells the unit council chair his idea for standardization of gait belt location. The chair encourages John to complete a FLIGHT SBAR tool and submit for review and approval. The chair advises John that if he has questions about the SBAR to come to her and she will assist in completing. John completed the SBAR and submitted the request to the chair. In the SBAR, there were questions directing John to determine who the stakeholders were in the project and who he would suggest work with him on the project. John knew that physical therapy would be a stakeholder and advised, in the SBAR, that he felt a team of two (himself and a physical therapist) could complete the project in approximately three weeks. The chair reviewed the SBAR request with her coach and determined the project would fit into the bucket of improvement in a quality initiative (and reducing falls was an organizational goal), so the project was approved. The chair met with John to set the timeline for progression and the milestones that needed to be met for the project to be complete in three weeks. John and the chair determined the number of hours that both he and a physical therapist could use toward the project. The chair met weekly with John, now the project lead, to be kept apprised of the project's movement and to identify any barriers the project lead was experiencing. John was able to complete the project in the three-week defined goal. John felt encouraged that his idea was able to be realized and he had ownership in helping his peers understand why the project was important to him. Many of his peers stated that not having to search for gait belts was an improvement and something they wished they had thought of themselves. The chair, at the completion of the project, asked John to share the project at the next unit council chair meeting and the nursing leadership meeting. Although nervous to do so, John shared his project with both groups. He was surprised to find out that many other units also had the same problem with finding gait belts and wanted information about how to implement this process on their units. He felt empowered that his idea made a difference in promoting patient safety and improved team workflow.

Role Clarification

Role responsibility and accountability are fundamental for the success of the FLIGHT Model. A clear understanding of role expectations is necessary for creating accountability for the entire team. This model allows and encourages professional employees to develop as leaders. They do this by participating in process improvement, leading projects, collaborating with the interdisciplinary team, developing evidence-based practice, and improving outcomes. In this section you will find sample roles and the associated expectations for that role (see Table 3.1). These roles can be used as a starting point for establishing accountability for council and leadership team member role development for your unique organization.

TABLE 3.1 FLIGHT Team Role Delineations and Expectations

Project Team Lead	
Who Can Fill Role	Any interprofessional employee (e.g., registered nurse, aide, tech, pharmacist, physical therapist) who has an idea or who is willing to execute an idea that is important to him/her
Qualities Required	Team-focused
	Desire to make a difference
	Desire to build project management skills

continues

TABLE 3.1 FLIGHT Team Role Delineations and Expectations (cont.)

Expectations	Submits idea/concern/issue for consideration along with possible improvement solutions using the SBAR tool
	Owns the project once it has been selected and approved to begin
	Meets with the chair and coach to determine timeline and milestones
	Works with the chair and coach to determine number of project team members needed and selection of those members
	Collaborates with peers to support project development and sustainment
	Works within the approved project timeline and budget to address issue using the plan, do, study, act process and to monitor sustainability
	Logs hours spent on projects
Project Team Member	
Who Can Fill Role	Any interprofessional employee from the unit involved (both clinical and nonclinical)
Qualities Required	Team-focused
	Desire to make a difference
Expectations	Works with the project lead on a defined project for the duration of the project
	Logs hours spent on project
Unit Council Chair	
Who Can Fill Role	Clinical nurse from the unit
Qualities Required	Team-focused
	Is seen as a unit resource and informal leader
	Possesses basic project management skills (or willing to learn)
	Has a keen understanding of current unit-based issues

Expectations	Provides overarching management of all projects occurring on the unit
	Reviews employee SBAR submissions and works with coach and unit leadership to prioritize projects
	Assists project leads in formulating a project timeline and budgetary needs as well as forecasting possible project members
	Meets with project leads on a routine basis
	Helps recruit project team members, if needed
	Supports and monitors project status, timeline, and budget
	Reviews project records
	Presents project summaries to nursing leadership using a standardized unit council reporting tool
	Consults with coach and other leadership to address barriers encountered by project leads to coach and other nursing leadership as appropriate
	Attends organizational unit council chair/coach meetings
	Builds and supports your team

Unit Council Coach

Who Can Fill Role	Unit-based frontline leader (e.g., charge nurse, unit supervisor, assistant manager, manager)
Qualities Required	Utilizes previous and current experience to teach and mentor project management skills
	Ability to manage multiple projects at a time
	Communicates in a positive and constructive manner
	Ability and willingness to mentor the chair, project leads, and project members
Expectations	Supports the chair in all responsibilities listed for chair
	Meets routinely with the chair
	Communicates unit projects and status reports to other leaders
	Enlists assistance from colleagues to ensure success of projects
	Assists with communication plan for entire unit

continues

TABLE 3.1   FLIGHT Team Role Delineations and Expectations (cont.)

Expectations (cont.)	Removes barriers as identified by project leads/members or the chair
	Ensures privacy and regulatory compliance
	Maintains knowledge of employees' participation as project lead and/or member for inclusion in annual review process
	Attends organizational unit council chair/coach meetings
	Builds and supports your team
Unit Leader (who is not the coach)	
Who Can Fill Role	Frontline leader (e.g., charge nurse, unit supervisor, assistant manager, manager)
Qualities Required	Guides direct reports to utilize the FLIGHT Model
	Communicates in a positive and constructive manner
	Mentors chair, project leads, and project members when coach is unavailable
Expectations	Supports project success and project leads
	Ensures communication regarding projects across all shifts
	Recruits project leads and project members
	Removes barriers as identified by project leads, members, or chair
	Ensures privacy and regulatory compliance
	Supports implementation and "go-live" aspects of project completion
	Maintains knowledge of employees' participation as project lead or member for inclusion in annual review process
	Builds and supports your team
Manager	
Who Can Fill Role	Unit- or division-level decision-maker
Qualities Required	Provides insight and perspective on upcoming issues and unit priorities
	Guides direct reports to utilize the FLIGHT Model
	Communicates in a positive and constructive manner
	Mentors chair, project leads, and project members

Expectations	Remains actively aware of all projects and requests project updates from the chair and coach on a routine basis
	Meets routinely with chair and coach
	Provides organizational perspective to unit projects (e.g., quality metrics, employee satisfaction survey results, patient satisfaction/experience survey results, themes from recent patient complaints)
	Reviews, with the chair and coach, proposed projects submitted through SBARs and assists in prioritizing them for future work
	Removes barriers as identified by the chair or coach
	Actively encourages and recruits unit employees for project lead, project member, unit council chair, and coach positions
	Assists in securing necessary resources to support a project's goals or a project's team lead (e.g., supplies, consultants)
	Provides a forum and a method for communication of projects (e.g., dedicated time at employee meetings, updates during shift huddles)
	Encourages celebration activities at completion of projects
	Builds and supports the team

Director or Executive Director	
Who Can Fill Role	Division or health system administrator
Qualities Required	Provides insight and perspective on upcoming issues and health system priorities
	Ability to guide direct reports to utilize the FLIGHT Model process
	Communicates in a positive and constructive manner
	Ability and willingness to mentor chair, project leads, project members, and manager

continues

TABLE 3.1   FLIGHT Team Role Delineations and Expectations (cont.)

Expectations	Performs all aspects as defined under manager role
	Promotes and highlights unit council projects and outcomes to the broader leadership team through structured presentations
	Meets with the manager, chair, and coach on a periodic basis
	Facilitates interdepartmental collaboration and cooperation as needed
	Ensures unit projects are in alignment with nursing and organizational goals
	Has ultimate authority for all project approval and for dispersal of resources to assist with project completion

It is imperative that all those supporting the FLIGHT Model have a clear understanding of what will be expected of them and how they can meet or exceed those expectations. We recommend sharing these expectations at unit council development sessions, employee meetings, and leadership meetings.

As in all matters pertaining to healthcare, communication is key. The FLIGHT Model will not be successful if there is insufficient communication about what is occurring on the unit level to those who are affected. It is important to communicate clearly to all unit employees (nursing and interprofessional team members) about:

- What projects are currently in flight
- What the status of those projects are
- Who the project lead is and what the anticipated go-live or implementation date is
- What projects are in the queue
- The method to ensure projects, once completed, are sustained

The FLIGHT Model further relies on both formal and informal avenues in which project leads, chairs, and coaches can report to the department's senior leaders (directors and managers) the work the council is doing, the roadblocks being experienced, and what support is needed to remove these roadblocks.

References

Attridge, M. (2009). Measuring and managing employee work engagement: A review of the research and business literature. *Journal of Workplace Behavioral Health, 24*(4), 383–398. doi: 10.1080/15555240903188398

Devi, V. R. (2009). Employee engagement is a two-way street. *Human Resource Management International Digest, 17*(2), 3–4. Retrieved from https://doi.org/10.1108/09670730910940186

Mattson, D. (2017, November 21). *The importance of communication between managers and their team.* Retrieved from https://www.sandler.com/blog/importance-communication-between-managers-and-their-team

Maxwell, J. C. (2001). *Team: The 17 indisputable laws of teamwork: Winning with people.* Nashville, TN: Thomas Nelson.

Mishra, K., Boynton, L., & Mishra, A. (2014). Driving employee engagement: The expanded role of internal communications [Abstract]. *International Journal of Business Communication, 51*(2). doi: 10.1177/2329488414525399

Wakeman, D. (2015, September 23). 3 Steps to align project and strategy. *Project Manager.* Retrieved from https://www.projectmanager.com/blog/3-steps-to-align-project-and-strategy

References

"Anytime you influence the thinking, beliefs, or development of another person, you're engaging in leadership."

–Ken Blanchard and Mark Miller

4

DEFINING LEADERSHIP: WHAT IT TAKES TO LEAD TODAY

General Characteristics of Leadership

What is a leader? There are volumes of books, articles, and journals devoted just to this topic. There are models, theories, and opinions. But for this book, we define a "leader" as an individual who works with others to develop a clear vision of the preferred future and to make that happen. We distinguish between those who hold a clear leadership (or management) title and those who are "leaders" regardless of what title or set of credentials they have behind their name.

Simply stated, leaders bring out the best in others. The ability and enthusiasm of unit-level managers and senior executives is crucial to the success of implementing models like the FLIGHT Model. The FLIGHT Model encourages and develops clinical nurses and others as leaders on their unit—but the support and mentoring of the formal leader for the unit is crucial. As discussed in Chapter 1, shared governance means sharing decision-making with frontline employees and management. Each has a unique and expert viewpoint that, when combined, allows for wise and successful decisions. Alone, each group is prone to silo thinking and can therefore make decisions that, in the end, do not always make the most sense. The American Organization of Nurse Executives (AONE) describes the link that nurse leaders provide between organizational objectives, daily operations, patient outcomes, and employee growth and experience:

> Nurse leaders with 24-hour accountability and responsibility for a
> direct care unit or units provide the vital link between the admin-
> istrative strategic plan and the point of care. The nurse manager is
> responsible for creating safe, healthy environments that support the
> work of the health care team and contribute to patient engagement.
> The role is influential in creating a professional environment and
> fostering a culture where interdisciplinary team members are able
> to contribute to optimal patient outcomes and grow professionally.
> (AONE, 2015, p. 3)

These leaders, for the purposes of this book, will be called managers. According to Marshall and Broome (2017) "leaders are seldom born, made, or found by luck, but rather emerge when preparation, character, experience, and circumstance come together at a time of need" (p. 15). Those leaders build on the strong leadership characteristics they always had. Leaders are most often ordinary people demonstrating extraordinary courage, skill, and "spirit to make a significant difference" (Kouzes & Posner, 2007, p. xiv).

When exploring predictive success factors for implementation of the FLIGHT Model, four attributes top the list. Specifically:

- Leadership style
- The ability to communicate and hold effective dialogues
- The effective use of power
- The ability and willingness to mentor

Leadership Style

In a study published in *The Journal of Nursing Administration* (Manning, 2016), three nurse manager leadership styles were studied in relation to clinical nurse work engagement: transformational, transactional, and passive-avoidant. Table 4.1 provides a description of each of these leadership styles.

TABLE 4.1   Leadership Styles

Leadership Style	Leader Characteristics
Transformational	Builds trust and confidence through personal association
	Develops a collective sense of mission and values
	Creates a collective vision
	Teaches and coaches on an individual basis
	Encourages innovation through examination and analysis of critical assumptions
Transactional	Provides meaningful rewards based upon task completion
	Seeks deviation from expectations and provides punishment
Passive-avoidant	Reacts to situations after they become serious
	Fails to lead

(Manning, 2016, p. 439)

This study determines that nurse manager leadership styles and clinical nurse work engagement were consistent with previous research findings. It suggests that a transformational leadership style positively influences clinical nurse work engagement. Manning (2016) concludes that:

> this positive impact on staff nurse work engagement may be explained through the supportive and relational leadership behaviors associated with transformational leadership styles. Examples of supportive leadership behaviors include role modeling, promoting a clear vision, innovation, creativity, and encouraging autonomy. (p. 442)

She further concludes that findings from the study support the importance of the leader communicating with followers, especially utilizing frequent feedback.

Because transactional leaders use their position power to either acknowledge or punish behavior, this leadership style does not complement the FLIGHT Model. Additionally, the passive-avoidant leadership style does not complement the FLIGHT Model. These leaders take a hands-off approach, delay decisions, provide no feedback, and make very little effort to satisfy the needs of followers.

The FLIGHT Model is best suited for use in organizations or within units or departments where the manager utilizes a transformational leadership style.

> Transformational leaders inspire others to achieve what might be considered extraordinary results. Leaders and followers engage with each other, raise each other, and inspire each other. Transformational leadership includes value systems, emotional intelligence, and attention to each individual's spiritual side. It connects with the very soul of the organization and honors its humanity. (Marshall & Broome, 2017, p. 15)

To be considered a transformational leader, you must choose to lead. This needs to be a conscious decision. Many excellent and competent nurses are given opportunities to supervise or manage, but successful leaders *choose* to lead. Some love the experience of leading and choose to continue this journey and become transformational leaders. Others determine that perhaps leadership is not where their talent, energy, or passion exists (Marshall & Broome, 2017). The beauty of the FLIGHT Model for unit-based professional governance centers on this very theme. Transformational managers will role-model transformational leadership in action, allowing clinical nurses the opportunity to "try their wings" in a bite-sized leadership role. The ability to self-discover talents and skills in a nonthreatening manner encourages the makings of more transformational leaders.

Five Practices of Transformational Leadership

Kouzes and Posner (2007, 2010) identify five practices in transformational leadership:

1. **Challenging the process,** which involves questioning the way things have been done in the past and thinking creatively about new solutions to old problems.

2. **Inspiring shared vision,** or bringing everyone together to move toward a goal that all accept as desirable and achievable.

3. **Enabling others to act,** which includes empowering people to believe that their extra effort will have rewards and will make a difference.

4. **Modeling the way,** meaning that the leader must take an active role in the work of change.

5. **Encouraging the heart,** by giving attention to those personal things that are important to people, such as saying "thank you" for a job well done and offering praise after a long day.

These practices are evident in the FLIGHT Model. Leaders are encouraged to question the status quo and to find solutions to problems. Once a possible solution is identified, leaders are asked to inspire others to bring a team together that can achieve the stated objective. The FLIGHT Model empowers all team members, regardless of credential or title, to have dedicated time to work on projects, thus enabling the process of change. The chair/coach dyad supports and models the way, providing an active role in the change. Finally, the FLIGHT Model is structured to provide encouragement from the heart through recognition pathways.

Communication and Dialogue

In addition to leadership styles, the FLIGHT Model is best utilized in organizations and on units where managers understand the importance of communication and have committed to promoting teamwork, collegiality, and maintaining an environment supportive of creative thinking and innovation. Unfortunately, communicating effectively sounds simple but is actually very difficult to operationalize. Table 4.2 shows the complexity of communication methods within an organization.

TABLE 4.2   Horizontal vs. Vertical Communication

	Horizontal Communication Style	Vertical Communication Style
Definition	Flow of information that occurs between persons holding the same position in the organization	Flow of information that occurs between superior and subordinates
Purpose	To coordinate activities of various departments and divisions of the organization	To provide necessary orders, instructions, and directives to the subordinates in downward direction; and receive suggestions, opinion, and feedback from the subordinates in an upward direction
Information flow	Between people holding the same rank and status	From superior to subordinates and vice versa
Degree of formality	Informal	Formal
Method of communication	Mostly through oral media	Mostly through written media
Possibility of distortion	Usually free from distortion	May suffer from distortion
Length of communication line	Short line: communication occurs between sender and receiver	Long line of communication

(adapted from The Business Communication, 2013, para. 3)

The complexities of healthcare, the varying audiences and levels of skill mix, and the sheer amount of information that needs to be shared can feel overwhelming. To mitigate these barriers, nursing managers often resort to a communication style that is autocratic, directive, and one-way. This style is efficient and comfortable for many who were raised and groomed in hierarchical organizations where this was standard practice. However, this one-way style often stunts a team's energy, creativity, learning, and results (Leebov & Scott, 2002).

The FLIGHT Model supports a work culture where information, perceptions, feelings, and ideas flow freely; where people express themselves and respect each other's viewpoints; and where all team members, colleagues, and stakeholders speak up for the good of the team and the mission. It supports a culture of engagement and values the varied perspectives and talents of all members of a team. This type of culture can only be realized if a team's formal leadership team is skilled in the art of dialogue and two-way communication. Dialogue, in contrast to one-way communication, draws people in as stakeholders in decisions and plans. When people engage in dialogue, they hear and retain more information, and the group comes to share responsibility for communication. When managers are skilled in dialogue and foster open, honest communication, they are valuable members of the team, have built trust and credibility, and are able to capitalize on everyone's thinking (Leebov & Scott, 2002).

Effective Use of Power

Power is the ability to exert influence, either formally or informally. According to Marshall and Broome (2017):

> Power is key to leadership. It is its underlying energy. To be an effective leader, you must become comfortable with power. There is power of position, power of personality, power in presence or of charisma, power of informal authority, and power by relationships with others of greater power. Power is the ability to move others, to move causes forward, and to extend both energy and assurance or confidence. It emanates from conviction, drive, and confidence in self; from a greater self; and from the direction of the organization. (p. 158)

In the book *Transformational Leadership in Nursing,* Marshall and Broome (2017, p. 159) outline the following attributes of a leader to acquire and sustain a strategic power base as delineated by Pfeffer:

- High energy and physical endurance, including the ability and motivation to personally contribute long and sometimes grueling hours to the work of the organization

- Directing energy to focus on clear strategic objectives, with attention to logistical details embedded within the objectives

- Successfully reading the behavior of others to understand key players, including the ability to assess willingness and resistance to following the leader's direction

- Adaptability and flexibility to redirect energy, abandon a course of action that is not working, and manage emotional responses to such situations

- Motivation to confront conflict, willingness to face difficult issues, and the ability to challenge difficult people to execute a successful strategic decision

- Subordinating the personal ego to the collective good of the organization by exercising discipline, restraint, and humility

Mentoring Future Leaders

There are multiple approaches that can be used to cultivate new leaders, but one of the most foundational is mentoring. Leaders who mentor have an instinctive *generativity*—a "concern in establishing and guiding the next generation" (Erikson, 1963, p. 267).

Marshall and Broome (2017) discuss the importance of mentoring:

> the transformational leader in health care has a constant eye on and heart for the next generation of leaders. To assure that any culture of practice excellence is sustained, leaders must habitually look beyond the present-day items at hand and focus on developing the leaders of tomorrow. (p. 264)

According to Marshall and Broome (2017, pp. 265–266), some key competencies and skills that effective mentors exhibit include:

- **Ability to develop a trusting mentoring relationship:** Mentoring is shared; thus, both the mentor and the mentee are responsible for creating a successful relationship.

- **Ability to advocate and provide opportunities:** Opening doors can be very impactful for a clinical nurse to develop new leadership skills and to gain visibility.

- **Ability to guide and counsel:** As the relationship develops over time, the mentor can be used to help understand conflict and various ways to deal with it—particularly when holding a leadership role.

- **Ability to teach:** Teaching involves not only imparting knowledge but also sharing personal experiences. Personal stories can be effective. Share the passion and drama of your leadership experiences, how you failed and learned from the failure, what your successes were, and how you learned to survive.

- **Ability to model:** Shadowing can be a great benefit to future leaders. Be profoundly aware of your own behavior, for you are always teaching by example.

- **Ability to motivate, inspire, and encourage:** Positive reinforcement along with affirmation of leadership abilities is crucial in developing their confidence.

- **Ability to challenge:** After a trusting relationship exists, challenging can occur by posing thought-provoking questions that allow self-reflection or different options/solutions. Encouraging them to take charge of a project and providing them with the resources is another way to challenge.

The FLIGHT Model encourages and supports each of these mentoring experiences and will be discussed in future chapters.

The Clinical Nurse as a Leader at the Bedside

Clinical nurses practicing at the bedside may believe their skill and ability in performing clinical procedures are what makes them appear professional to others (patients, families, peers, supervisors). If asked, they may say that leading and managing are skills and traits left to those in formal leadership roles. However, clinical nurses evidence leadership and management skills daily through assignment making, patient and family problem-solving, discharge planning, patient education, and coaching and mentoring employees (Yoder-Wise, 2007). Yoder-Wise identified the attributes that add to the credibility and capability of nurses as leaders and managers. Successful leaders and managers:

- "Use focused energy and stamina to accomplish a vision
- Use critical-thinking skills in decision-making
- Trust intuition, then back up intuition with facts
- Accept responsibility willingly and follow up on the consequences of actions taken
- Identify the needs of others
- Deal with people skillfully: coaches, communicates, counsels
- Demonstrate ease in standard boundary setting
- Examine multiple options to accomplish the objective at hand flexibly
- Are trustworthy and handle information from various sources with respect for the source
- Motivate others assertively toward the objective at hand
- Demonstrate competence or are capable of rapid learning in the arena where change is desired" (2007, p. 9)

In addition to attributes, effective teams have leaders (at all levels) that interchangeably practice leading, managing, and following. Table 4.3 delineates each of these tasks.

TABLE 4.3 The Tasks of Leading, Managing, and Following

Tasks of Leading	Tasks of Managing	Tasks of Following
Envision goals	Identify systems and processes	Recognize how individual responsibilities fit into organizational systems
Affirm values	Verify minimum and optimum standards/specifications	Honor the standards and specifications
Motivate	Validate the knowledge, skills, and abilities of available employees	Offer knowledge, skills, and abilities
Manage, including: Planning and priority setting Organizing and institution-building Keeping the system functioning Setting agendas and making decisions Exercising political judgment	Devise and communicate a comprehensive "big picture" plan	Collaborate willingly with leaders and managers
Achieve workable unity	Eliminate barriers/obstacles to work effectiveness	Include data collection as part of daily work activities
Develop trust	Measure the equity of workload	Demonstrate accountability for individual actions
Explain	Offer rewards and recognition to individuals and teams	Take reasonable risks
Serve as symbol	Recommend ways to improve systems and processes	Give feedback on the efficiency and effectiveness of systems
Represent the group	Involve others in decision-making	Give and receive feedback to and from other team members, leaders, and managers
Renew		

(Yoder-Wise, 2007, p. 23)

The FLIGHT Model of unit-based professional governance supports nurses at all levels to perform tasks around leading, managing, and following. It allows clinical nurses opportunities to lead projects, be a team member on a project, or be a responsible member of the greater population experiencing change. This allows active participation in developing and shaping policy and practices that affect patient care, the culture of the organization, and the work environment. The FLIGHT Model understands and promotes the inherent leadership skills that clinical nurses possess and provides a structure that encourages further development.

The FLIGHT Model supports projects of any size. Often employees begin their journeys by completing a small unit council project with success. With their realized success and their added confidence, they often will tackle a larger project later. With every project, employees experience the project workflow, develop their leadership skills, and learn the intricacies of leading through change. Without even realizing it, the FLIGHT Model provides employees with leadership skills that enable them to develop professionally and advance their careers when they are ready. Many project leads have been subsequently promoted to advanced positions, and many unit council chairs have accepted formal leadership positions on their units.

References

American Organization of Nurse Executives. (2015). *AONE nurse manager competencies.* Chicago, IL: Author. Retrieved from www.aone.org

The Business Communication. (2013, November 30). Differences between horizontal and vertical communication [Web log post]. Retrieved from https://thebusinesscommunication. com/differences-between-horizontal-and-vertical-communication/

Erikson, E. H. (1963). *Childhood and society* (2nd ed.). New York, NY: Norton.

Kouzes, J. M., & Posner, B. Z. (2007). *The leadership challenge* (4th ed.). San Francisco, CA: Jossey-Bass.

Kouzes, J. M., & Posner, B. Z. (2010). *The five practices of exemplary leadership* (2nd ed.). Hoboken, NJ: John Wiley & Sons.

Leebov, W., & Scott, G. (2002). *The indispensable health care manager: Success strategies for a changing environment.* San Francisco, CA: Jossey-Bass.

Manning, J. (2016). The influence of nurse manager leadership style on staff nurse work engagement. *JONA, 46*(9), 438–443. doi: 10.1097/NNA.0000000000000372

Marshall, E. S., & Broome, M. E. (2017). *Transformational leadership in nursing: From expert clinician to influential leader* (2nd ed.). New York, NY: Springer Publishing Company, LLC.

Yoder-Wise, P. S. (2007). *Leading and managing in nursing* (4th ed.). St. Louis, MO: Mosby Elsevier.

"The focus of gap analysis should be getting to the other side. If you bend over to analyze a gap too long, you'll probably fall into it."

–Ryan Lilly

5

PRE-FLIGHT ASSESSMENT: IDENTIFYING THE NEED FOR CHANGE

Current State Analysis and Opportunities for Change

We used "current state–ideal state" methodology to help us crystalize our thinking when developing the FLIGHT Model. This methodology required asking task force members to identify what was currently in place, including what was working well and what was not working well. The members then brainstormed what an ideal state would be. What the team really needed was a tool to measure the gap between the current state moving to the ideal state.

When assessing your organizational readiness, evaluation of the advantages and disadvantages of a change warrant consideration. Advantages of the FLIGHT Model include leadership development of clinical employees, empowering and engaging employees, and a foundation that ensures all members of the team and leadership are working toward common organizational objectives. The areas we suggest you assess in your current state include:

- Power gradient, equity, and workplace violence
- Project alignment with strategic goals
- Leadership engagement
- Return on investment (ROI): projects, meetings, and unit-based teams
- The existence of interprofessional teams
- Establishment and utilization of communication channels
- Shared accountability for outcomes
- Existence of support systems for unit-based projects and frontline leaders
- Employee satisfaction
- Unit and employee engagement in improvement efforts
- Establishment of shift worker participation

Odds are, if you're reading this book, you are likely searching for an improvement in your current unit-based structure. This model is not a cookie cutter model that can simply be applied to your current organizational state and produce ideal outcomes. It is important for you and your leadership team to complete a readiness gap analysis and validate if your current state and your ideal state (full implementation of the FLIGHT Model) are aligned. If alignment is clear, adopting the concepts of the FLIGHT Model could be easily integrated. If your current state is far removed from your ideal state, there will be both cultural and structural work for you and your teams to do before undertaking implementation of the FLIGHT Model.

According to Couto, Plansky, and Caglar (2017):

> Change ... must be grounded in the organization's culture. Those on the front line and in the back office [must] embrace and enable the change, and the only way that will happen is if you leverage what works in your company's culture ... To get people to come on board and stay on board with the new normal, you [must] enlist your culture—the intangible collections of instinctive, repetitive habits and emotional cues and responses that determine what people feel, think, and believe about their work. (p. 28)

It might be overwhelming to think about all the necessary change. Kotter and Rathgeber (2005) suggest that using a systematic process to design change allows leaders to plan success. Kotter and Rathgeber (2005) explain the importance of creating a sense of urgency to help others on the team understand the need for change, developing a team to make it happen, initiating and implementing the change, and supporting a culture to maintain the changes long term.

Completing a Current State Gap Analysis

In the next section of this chapter you will have the opportunity to complete a gap analysis on topics that help you identify the current state of your organizational readiness, leadership readiness, and employee readiness. The tool built at the end of this section will help identify gaps and help you and your team develop a sense of urgency while clearly defining opportunity areas for growth. The self-analysis section and tool are designed to assess your:

1. Organizational readiness

2. Leadership readiness

3. Employee readiness

Organizational Readiness: Evaluate the Power Gradient/Equity in Your Organization

Power, control, and equity are real in the workplace, and some may even say heightened in the healthcare setting. Workplace violence in the form of bullying is becoming more evident in research, and while partner violence and workplace violence differ, they often have common abusive characteristics (Scott, 2018):

- **Intimidation:** Instilling fear by behavior, including looks, acts, and gestures

- **Coercion:** Making threats to team members, including unjustified punishment or loss of employment

- **Isolation:** This can occur when someone controls contact with colleagues or limits access to information, using pretended support or concern to justify actions

- **Economic abuse:** Denying financial rewards, or barring promotion

- **Emotional abuse:** Persistent humiliation, name-calling, unwanted jokes, or playing mind games

Abuse of power and control when exerted in the workplace often has a negative impact on job-related duties and overall health such as mental disorientation, physical health problems, symptoms of post-traumatic stress, burnout, increased intentions to leave, reduced job satisfaction, and reduced commitment to the organization (Nielsen & Einarsen, 2012). When assessing readiness for your department or workplace, it is important to recognize these behaviors. If the behaviors are widespread, consider developing an action plan to eliminate workplace violence or workplace bullying prior to initiating any model of employee engagement or change. Figure 5.1 illustrates that power and control wheel modified for workplace bullying.

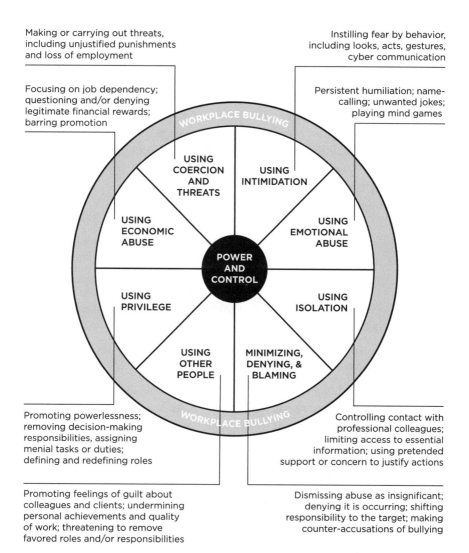

Making or carrying out threats, including unjustified punishments and loss of employment

Instilling fear by behavior, including looks, acts, gestures, cyber communication

Focusing on job dependency; questioning and/or denying legitimate financial rewards; barring promotion

Persistent humiliation; name-calling; unwanted jokes; playing mind games

Promoting powerlessness; removing decision-making responsibilities, assigning menial tasks or duties; defining and redefining roles

Controlling contact with professional colleagues; limiting access to essential information; using pretended support or concern to justify actions

Promoting feelings of guilt about colleagues and clients; undermining personal achievements and quality of work; threatening to remove favored roles and/or responsibilities

Dismissing abuse as insignificant; denying it is occurring; shifting responsibility to the target; making counter-accusations of bullying

FIGURE 5.1 Workplace bullying wheel.
(Scott, 2018)

Organizational Readiness: Evaluate Project Alignment in Current State

Frontline or unit-based decision-making teams may have a difficult time tying projects to the organization's strategic plan. Leaders considering the adoption of the FLIGHT Model should critically evaluate whether current unit-based improvement projects and completed previous projects match or sync with the organizational plan. It is common for a unit-based project to be deployed in a silo without necessarily aligning with the larger organization's strategic plans. Some important questions to ask your teams include:

- What process does our team use to prioritize projects as high or low?
- How does our group balance projects that focus on improving quality, safety, and employee satisfaction?
- Do we have a requirement for pre- and post-data collection?
- Has our leadership team provided tools for project management, strategy, and implementation?
- Have we shared the organization's strategic plan with the team, and have we tasked our team to focus on a specific goal?

This evaluation is focused on validating that you have a systematic process that supports unit-level teams to select and utilize resources that allow teams to maximize value (Sifri, 2008). It is common for teams considering the FLIGHT Model to find that unit-level projects do not tie back to or align with the organization's strategic plan.

Organizational Readiness: Leadership Engagement in Current Structure

Leadership engagement is essential when analyzing optimal readiness. We recommend you ask an important question—"Am I a change agent?" The FLIGHT Model is closely dependent on a person's or a leadership team's ability to lead or inspire change. A useful method for assessing leadership engagement or readiness is assessing your leadership values. Leaders who have clear values often have a strong voice, can express their ideas and direction, make tough decisions, are determined, and take charge rather than imitating others (Kouzes & Posner, 1987). Characteristics to evaluate when assessing leader readiness include (Kouzes & Posner, 1987):

- A positive sense of team spirit
- A sense of organizational pride
- A willful and deep commitment to your team and organization
- Strong motivation
- Strong feelings to make a difference
- Strong levels of trust with your team

Having the right leaders participate in early adoption efforts is key to FLIGHT success. It is difficult or impossible for employees to be engaged unless the leader is actively engaged (Kerfoot, 2007). If you and your team agree that you and your leadership hold several of the attributes described above, your self-assessment could indicate one phase of readiness for adoption of the FLIGHT Model.

Organizational Readiness: Evaluate "Bang for Your Buck" in Current State

In this environment you need to be able to show bang for your buck. This evaluation will not take hours of your time. You will not need to run budget reports or meet with executive leaders. Your evaluation of ROI can be completed simply by considering some of the work you have recently done during your evaluation phase.

Take a moment to consider several previous and current projects your teams are or have been working on. You should have an active focus on (Cohen, Ptaskiewicz, & Mipos, 2010):

- Clinical outcomes
- Operations
- Patient benefits
- Interdisciplinary involvement

As a leader, you may have background knowledge on the relationship between high employee engagement and high performance. This should be considered when evaluating your ROI in group work. Cohen et al.'s (2010) research suggests that highly engaged employees are twice as likely to become high performers; they often exceed performance expectations and easily relate to the organization and its customer. As you consider your current ROI, can you easily identify your impact on clinical outcomes, daily and long-term operations, patient benefits, and involvement of different workforce team members?

It is also important to gather some basic facts about the cost of your current meeting structure. Several online tools exist to calculate the cost of a meeting. Let's review the cost of a monthly four-hour meeting using average salaries for a multidisciplinary team (Bureau of Labor Statistics, US Department of Labor, n.d.):

- Three frontline nurses ($68,450/year)
- One charge nurse ($59,380/year)
- One nursing assistant ($26,419/year)

According to the *Harvard Business Review* (2016), this meeting will cost $840 for four hours per month, which translates to an annual cost of $10,080. At the end of this four-hour meeting, if you have not affected clinical outcomes or operations, improved patient care, or increased engagement, what do you have as an ROI for your investment in the traditional model of unit-based governance?

Leadership Readiness: Evaluate Interprofessional Involvement in Projects

Interprofessional teamwork refers to a group of different healthcare professionals delivering patient-centered care that is highly collaborative and well-coordinated (Eggenberger, Sherman, & Keller, 2014). The work of creating an interprofessional team is always intentional, and a leader's role in developing this team is helping the team move past daily duties, conflicts, and poor communication while developing a common goal that improves patient outcomes (Eggenberger et al., 2014). Leaders evaluating interprofessional involvement can assess unit-level work groups and project outputs using the following questions:

- Do you have a unit-based interprofessional team that is not your rounding team?
- What projects has your interprofessional team worked on together?

- How have you supported the success of this team?
- Do you have measurable data from your interprofessional team that supports quality, safety, or engagement?

A positive correlation of interprofessional involvement will have clear and intentional team development, communication, and synergy while speaking highly toward your readiness to implement the FLIGHT Model.

Leadership Readiness: Evaluate Communication Channels

Successful unit-based teams utilize all available communication channels for two-way messaging. As a leader evaluating communication streams and the current state of frontline project success, you will want to consider:

- Does your program have built-in educational streams?
  - Fundamental project management skill sessions
  - Coaching
  - Open and available seminars
- Do you have a path for successful projects to be shared with a larger group or team?
- When your team is lost or off track, do you or other leaders intervene before momentum is lost?
- Do you have a formal mentoring and coaching plan for unit-based leaders and project managers? If not, do these unit-based leaders have access to others skilled in project management?
  - Can your unit-based leaders approach these resources independently?
- Have you established a sounding board or venue for project leaders to learn from each other?

This evaluation is crucial for supporting the success of developing projects that support your organization's strategic plan. Unit-based project leaders need a clear path for both vertical and horizontal communication.

Horizontal and vertical communication are essential for team success. Horizontal communication is important as it supports peer-to-peer and department-level communication. Horizontal communication is great for co-ordination and sharing of ideas. Vertical communication may be more formal than horizontal, but it supports leadership and employee communication, collaboration, and support (The Business Communication, 2018). Vertical communication helps bridge across the division or organization, thus reducing incidence of employees working in silos, which in turn supports project efficiency. And, most importantly, vertical communication helps to ensure all players on the team are working toward the same overall organizational objectives.

FLIGHT Simulator: Leadership in Action

A unit-based decision-making group meets bimonthly to share ideas, projects, and outcomes, utilizing a horizontal communication strategy. As this decision-making group developed over time, several members of nursing leadership began attending to provide organizational updates and offer suggestions while also listening to ideas, receiving feedback on current initiatives, and hearing frontline issues and opportunities for improvement.

This group had a specific purpose of exchanging horizontal information (peer-to-peer) and then matured to value leadership input and dialogue exchange, resulting in vertical information sharing.

Leadership Readiness: Evaluate Accountability of Outcomes

Unit-based teams must feel a sense of urgency and ownership to successfully lead projects that align with the organization's strategic plan. Leaders need to consciously strive to develop their teams by creating more leaders and move team members from dependence to independence and even interdependence. Leaders should help teams move toward (Ohlinger, Brown, Laudert, Swanson, & Fofah, 2003):

- Directing
- Coaching

- Supporting
- Delegating

When evaluating your team for outcomes, analyze your team's ability to direct projects, coach, provide peer-to-peer feedback, provide ample amounts of support, and, if appropriate, delegate tasks. Teams that are committed to improving unit-based outcomes often feel a sense of ownership as a whole, rather than a single leader owning outcomes independently. When considering your team's accountability, consider common goals among your unit, unit leaders, and project groups.

Leadership Readiness: Evaluate the Support System for Unit-Based Projects and Leaders

Unit-based projects and the leads of those projects need strategic support to provide positive output. This support varies from team to team based on project management skill level and knowledge. As you evaluate your current system for unit-based projects and leaders, you need to consider the following:

- Do your unit-based leaders approach you or the leadership team for direction and guidance?
- Do you have a list of resources so when team members get "lost" they know whom to seek out for guidance?
  - Quality leaders
  - Research development professionals
  - Project management guidance
- Do you provide ongoing education to your team for lifelong learning and support?
- Do you mentor your unit-based project leaders?
- Have you or the leadership team set individual goals for unit-based leaders?
- Do you have a clear expectation for your unit-based project teams?
- Do you have concurrent projects in employee engagement, quality, and safety (rather than a single project focus)?

As a leader, it will serve you well to take intentional steps to validate and verify that a solid and well-rounded support system for unit-based leaders is in place.

Employee Readiness: Evaluate Employee Satisfaction Results

Choose several of your departments and evaluate overall employee satisfaction. Do you have employee comments that ask for improvement, want the ability to offer ideas, or seek support or direction? These are good indicators that your movement toward the FLIGHT Model is heading in the right direction. When evaluating employee satisfaction, the emphasis should not solely rely on survey results but include other performance indicators such as (Crebar, 2016):

- The use of an employee suggestion box

- Employee engagement surveys

- Employee net promoter scores

- Employee absenteeism and turnover rate

Employee suggestion boxes play a vital role in maintaining high levels of satisfaction. Crebar's (2016) research suggests that these boxes help demonstrate to your employees that their voice and opinion matters while promoting change and increasing motivation and satisfaction. When analyzing your employee engagement, especially if you already utilize this tool, it is important to determine how readily it is used. Is the suggestion box ever used? If not, this would indicate that your team believes that shared opinions will not be taken seriously and ideas for improvement will not be implemented.

When evaluating employee surveys to measure engagement, it is important to seek honest feedback to accurately measure how valued employees feel, how satisfied they are with their work/life balance, and to explore feelings about career prospects (Crebar, 2016). If you have negative scores coming from your employee surveys, it is important to analyze whether adopting a program to improve engagement is the first step prior to implementing the FLIGHT Model.

Most employee engagement surveys contain employee net promoter scores that allow organizations to measure the levels of both satisfaction and loyalty by asking, "How likely would you recommend working here to a friend or colleague?" (Crebar, 2016). Positive overall scores reflect engaged employees, whereas low scores reflect an opportunity for growth.

Lastly, you will want to evaluate overall employee absenteeism and turnover rates; however, this is a lagging indicator. High rates of poor attendance and turnover often are a reflection that certain leaders or departments need additional attention to improve the employee experience (Crebar, 2016).

Employees Readiness: Engagement in Improvement Efforts

Measuring unit-level and employee engagement readiness may appear to be challenging initially. When units maintain high levels of engagement, it is often palpable. When attempting to do a pulse check on engagement, walk through the department(s) you are completing this assessment for and determine if you can feel the levels of (Kerfoot, 2007):

- Friendliness of the team
- Ambiance of happiness
- Attention to and quality of work
- Pride in unit
- Pride in organization

Unit-level and employee engagement are often a reflection of the unit leadership (Kerfoot, 2007). As a leader committed to analyzing your unit's or employee's readiness, using this technique during walking rounds will prepare you to analyze change readiness. As a leader preparing to introduce a new model that affects project output, you may also want to assess your department's previous and current frontline projects. Meet with frontline leaders and employees and actively investigate previous projects, the current state, and immediate past outcomes. Simultaneously assess the volume of current and upcoming projects.

This assessment will provide insight on what works and what does not while providing insight on your team's current level of engagement.

FLIGHT Simulator: Leadership in Action

On a 26-bed dialysis and metabolic unit that has approximately 70 employees, a nurse manager is actively preparing to analyze their unit's readiness to change and adopt the FLIGHT Model. The manager plans meetings with three of the unit-based leaders (assistant managers, charge nurses, etc.) and the unit council chair and chair.

The manager meets one-on-one with the assistant managers (or charge nurses, etc.) and asks the following very targeted questions:

- Can you tell me about our previous and current unit-based projects?
- What was your role?
- How was this introduced to you?
- How did you manage the project, timeline, milestones, and goals?
- How did you sustain these projects?
- How do you feel about learning a new project management style?
- How would your team describe you as the leader of projects?

Answers to these questions help guide the gap you and your team need to bridge in order to proceed with change.

Next, the manager meets with the established unit council chair and coach to assess their readiness. The manager asks targeted questions closely aligned to those of the assistant manager but adds team-building questions:

- Can you tell me about our previous and current unit-based projects?
- What was your role?
- How was this introduced to you?
- How did you manage the project, timeline, milestones, and goals?
- How did you sustain these projects?

- How do you feel about learning a new project management style?
- How do you feel about asking more team members to participate in improving our department?
- What do you love most about our department?
- What ideas do you currently have to improve our department?
- As a team, do you think we can implement change to improve some of those ideas?
- Can you see yourself leading a project that improves our department?
- If we start a project next week, could you possibly find three more team members to participate?

A forthright discussion around these topics for both frontline leaders and chairs will drive your decision on whether the unit is ready to participate in adopting the FLIGHT Model.

Employee Readiness: Evaluate Projects Arising From Off-Shifts

Acute care centers are 24/7 and have employees that cover up to four shifts. A robust unit-based team will have projects and outcomes that improve quality, safety, and engagement on all shifts.

FLIGHT Simulator: Leadership in Action

In a 34-bed post-surgical unit, a team of night shift employees asked a unit-based leader if there was something they could do to improve the discharge process. The leader took a moment to think and realized this team could improve the after-visit summary (AVS) containing next dose times, clinical references, and nursing notes for discharge.

Two night shift nurses took the idea and met with day shift nurses to come up with a 24-hour discharge preparation workflow. The night shift nurses received education on completing the electronic portion of the after-visit summary by working elbow to elbow with the discharging employees.

The night shift nurses then designed a survey to collect pre- and post-assessment data related to workflow improvements when discharging a patient. After the pre-assessment data was collected, the two night shift nurses trained all night shift employees on completing several areas of the AVS. A go-live date was determined, and the team started the new process. The team had an immediate improvement in time needed to complete an AVS at the point of patient discharge.

This project had tremendous measurable success, and the two night shift nurses had an immense sense of pride in strategically improving quality and workflow in their departments.

The following tool is included in this book to help you perform a gap analysis for your unit or organization. It will help you determine your area's readiness for change.

TABLE 5.1   Gap Analysis Tool

Gap Analysis Tool			
Evaluation Criteria	**Met**	**Unmet**	**Comments**
The existence of power gradient/ equity/workplace violence Do I level the power gradient/equity/ workplace violence?			
Project alignment with strategic goals Do I help the team align projects with the system's strategic plan and goals?			

Leadership engagement Are my fellow leaders and I actively engaged in unit-based improvements?			
ROI on projects, meetings, and unit-based teams Is the ROI clear enough to the team and do we understand how the structure improves quality, safety, and engagement?			
The existence of interprofessional teams: clear projects and outcomes Is there an interprofessional team that participates in projects that improve quality, safety, and workflow?			
Established and utilized communication channels Do I create and support all communication channels that support unit-based decision-making?			
Shared accountability for outcomes Do we share accountability with frontline team members or is a single person accountable for goals?			
Existence of support systems for unit-based projects and frontline leaders Do I or our leaders have a clear structure for support and development?			
Employee satisfaction results Does the current state have positive employee satisfaction results?			

continues

TABLE 5.1 Gap Analysis Tool   (cont.)

Evaluation Criteria	Met	Unmet	Comments
Unit/employees engagement in improvement efforts Do the unit and employees take an active role in outcomes, safety, quality, and engagement?			
Establishment of shift worker participation in project and improvement Does the team have equal levels of participation from shift to shift?			
Total of overall Met and Unmet	**Total:**	**Total:**	

Identifying Current State Barriers and Planning for an Ideal State

Now that you have reflected on your current state and have identified areas of success and areas for improvement, it is time to focus on identifying the barriers that got you here. An evaluation that confirms a greater response in the "met" column suggests that your department, division, or organization may be ready for adoption of FLIGHT without major disruption. For an assessment or evaluation that has multiple or a majority of "unmet" responses, focus on starting an open dialogue with frontline teams and leaders, developing a road map to FLIGHT adoption, working toward improvements, and staying positive (see Figure 5.2). The following sections discuss the main characteristics you will need in order to remove barriers.

Have Open Dialogue

Using the results from the evaluation, develop talking points to use with leaders and frontline employees during rounds, employee meetings, and huddles. Starting dialogue with key stakeholders will allow you to meet with teams and individuals to discuss, share, and receive ideas on improvement.

Develop a Map

After this dialogue, you will want to take this feedback and develop a plan to achieve improvement. Since you are working toward FLIGHT, consider involving frontline employees and leaders in all levels of change. Focus strategically on incorporating employees to participate in all changes. Share your plan with the team and members you met with during your dialogue phase.

Work on Improvement

Having a constant focus on small improvements will provide huge wins and success for your team downstream. With a renewed energy that has a focus on two-way communication (both horizontal and vertical), you will surely create new avenues for frontline engagement.

Stay Positive

The outcomes of change are not always clear. You will need to measure specific metrics on surveys or through other means of data collection to evaluate the effectiveness of change. This type of growth and development is not quick, and at times it may become difficult designing and implementing sustained, positive change.

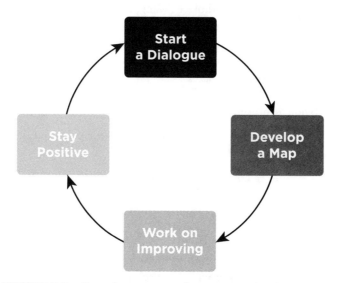

FIGURE 5.2 Ongoing process for overcoming barriers.

Success in removing barriers as you make your way toward an ideal state requires an ongoing, long-term commitment to keeping communication open, evaluating and updating the plan, and keeping morale high.

Additional Considerations When Completing a Gap Analysis

Several additional barriers exist that must be considered when completing your current state gap analysis, such as:

- The impact of a generational shift
- Rapid healthcare change
- Limited employee engagement
- Managerial relations

Impact of a Generational Shift

Acute care centers of any size have multigenerational workforces just by the nature of the required work and turnover. Each workforce generation has their own values and ways of completing assigned tasks and duties, but they are still required to share the same workplace (Wang, 2015). As a leader of a multigenerational workforce working to improve quality, safety, and engagement, you will need to leverage each team member or be stuck with teams that function poorly. Wang (2015) offers simple interventions and strategies to improve multigenerational barriers to success:

- Provide mentoring opportunities
  - Set up and manage opportunities for peer-to-peer mentoring conducted by specific generations.
    - For example: Allow millennials to teach technology-based skills while providing opportunities for baby boomers to share stories of skill and technique.
- Establish an equal voice
  - Set up forums or meetings that allow members of each generation to provide feedback or opinions. Creating this opportunity will allow your team to share a differing prospective while gaining insight into how their colleagues think.

The key to removing the multigenerational gap is providing options that meet the needs of the individual groups.

Rapid Change in Healthcare

Healthcare is changing at lightning speed, and with the adoption of data analytics into clinical practice, what we did yesterday is completely new and different today. But change and adoption of new technology, service lines, and product evolution are most closely related to loss; when change occurs, individuals and teams experience the loss of what was (Guerin, 2013). As change continues at a rapid rate, it is important to remember that someone on your team is most likely experiencing the change as a loss.

Limited Employee Engagement

Acute care centers are in operation 24 hours a day, 7 days a week. If you found in your evaluation that only the day shift is engaged, you will need to take proactive steps to engage other shifts. Some actions you can take include:

- Offer meetings in the evening
- Find a shift worker barrier and lead the team to a small success
- Offer mentoring on evening and night shifts

Managerial Relations

Managers play a vital role in removing barriers and improving employee engagement. Managers are considered gate-keepers in aligning organizational goals with frontline teams. Managers should focus on (Foster, 2017):

- **Setting clear objectives:** Set a clear and established goal for the entire team and determine how you will meet it.
- **Motivating people:** Motivate your team by providing the opportunity for others to be successful.
- **Positive communication:** Communicate early and effectively in a manner that meets the needs of your team.
- **Developing people:** Make your team valuable; teach skills, techniques, and mentor.

Your gap analysis evaluation may determine that a new urgency exists while much preparatory work lies ahead. The onus is on you, the manager, to take positive steps toward making improvements or changes that will lead to increased safety, quality, and employee engagement in your workplace. Your evaluation results will serve as the first step in making those improvements—now you know what areas are in need of change before you prepare to take flight. The next chapter will explore change theory and how it can be applied to the FLIGHT Model to ensure success.

References

Bureau of Labor Statistics, Unites States Department of Labor. (n.d.). *Occupational employment statistics: Occupational employment and wages, May 2017: 29-1141 registered nurses*. Retrieved from https://www.bls.gov/oes/current/oes291141.htm

The Business Communication. (2018, March 17). Differences between horizontal and vertical communication [Web log post]. Retrieved from https://thebusinesscommunication.com/differences-between-horizontal-and-vertical-communication/

Cohen, P. M., Ptaskiewicz, M., & Mipos, D. (2010). The case for unit-based teams: A model for frontline engagement and performance improvement. *The Permanente Journal, 14*(2). doi: 10.7812/tpp/09-126

Couto, V., Plansky, J., & Caglar, D. (2017). *Fit for growth: A guide to strategic cost cutting, restructuring, and renewal*. Hoboken, NJ: John Wiley and Sons.

Crebar, A. (2016, May 7). *4 KPIs to measure employee engagement*. Retrieved from https://www.saplinghr.com/blog/4-kpis-measure-employee-engagement

Eggenberger, T., Sherman, R. O., & Keller, K. (2014, November). Creating high-performance interprofessional teams. *American Nurse Today, 9*(11). Retrieved from https://www.americannursetoday.com/creating-high-performance-interprofessional-teams/

Foster, J. (2017, March 16). *The impact of managers on workplace engagement and productivity*. Retrieved from https://www.interact-intranet.com/blog/the-impact-of-managers-on-workplace-engagement-and-productivity/

Guerin, S. (2013, February 28). Managing rapid change in the health care environment. *Managed Care*. Retrieved from https://www.managedcaremag.com/archives/2013/2/managing-rapid-change-health-care-environment

Harvard Business Review. (2016, January 11). *Estimate the cost of a meeting with this calculator*. Retrieved from https://hbr.org/2016/01/estimate-the-cost-of-a-meeting-with-this-calculator

Kerfoot, K. (2007). Staff engagement: It starts with the leader. *Nursing Economic$, 37*(3), 28–29. Retrieved from https://annanurse.org/download/reference/update/Volume37_Issue3/pages28-29.pdf

Kotter, J. P., & Rathgeber. H. (2005). *Our iceberg is melting: Changing and succeeding under any conditions*. New York, NY: St. Martin's Press.

Kouzes, J. M., & Posner, B. Z. (1987). *The leadership challenge* (5th ed.). San Francisco, CA: Jossey-Bass.

Nielsen, M. B., & Einarsen, S. (2012). Outcomes of exposure to workplace bullying: A meta-analytic review. *Work & Stress, 26*(4), 309–332. doi: 10.1080/02678373.2012.734709

Ohlinger, J., Brown, M. S., Laudert, S., Swanson, S., & Fofah, O. (2003). Development of potentially better practices for the neonatal intensive care unit as a culture of collaboration: Communication, accountability, respect, and empowerment. *Pediatrics, 111*(4), 471–481. Retrieved from https://www.semanticscholar.org/paper/Development-of-potentially-better-practices-for-the-Ohlinger-Brown/59b4e37e2530f71318f145108cfaf4393f59a3cd

Scott, H. S. (2018). Extending the Duluth model to workplace bullying: A modification and adaptation of the workplace power-control wheel. *Workplace Health & Safety, 66*(9), 444–452. doi: 10.1177/2165079917750934

Sifri, G. (2008, November 18). Prioritize projects to align with strategic plan. *Tech Republic.* Retrieved from https://www.techrepublic.com/blog/tech-decision-maker/prioritize-projects-to-align-with-strategic-plan-116516/

Wang, D. (2015, January 8). *Don't let the generation gap threaten employee engagement.* Retrieved from https://www.tinypulse.com/blog/dont-let-the-generation-gap-threaten-employee-engagement

3

TAKING FLIGHT

"You never change things by fighting the existing reality. To change something, build a new model that makes the existing model obsolete."

–Buckminster Fuller

6

APPLYING CHANGE THEORY TO THE FLIGHT MODEL

- Understand the importance of selecting a change theorist prior to implementing the FLIGHT Model or other unit governance change
- Become familiar with change theories
- Describe how Kotter's Change Theory influences the FLIGHT Model
- Identify, through examples, the stages of change

The evolving healthcare environment is pushing organizations to be more innovative, adaptive, and creative in managing performance with the current pace of external change. Using a change management theory when implementing a new structure increases the opportunity for success. Using a change theory helps navigate your thoughts and actions as you plan, implement, and sustain the change. In this chapter we outline both the importance of understanding and planning for change as well as discuss various change theories.

Planning for Change

There are certain elements that must be in place prior to implementing change: the direction for change, an effective and functional leadership structure, and a culture that promotes and rewards change. The vision must be articulated clearly and communicated to everyone in the organization. It is important to continually reinforce the vision to foster a culture that is ready for the changes needed to move toward the goal (Gesme & Wiseman, 2010). Planned change does not occur without developing an agreed-upon goal; those involved in the vision could be leaders, employees, or ideally a combination of both.

In the development of the FLIGHT Model, the idea for a new approach to our unit council structure was proposed by a clinical nurse. It was then brought to a leader, and a team was formed with a combination of leaders and clinical employees. This group worked together to create a vision, and set attainable goals. By using this approach, we were able to tap into multiple perspectives, generate many ideas, and together form a shared vision. We recommend this team approach when planning and developing a new unit council structure in your organization.

In addition to a team, it is important to have functional and effective managers who understand, support, and are committed to the vision, and understand the work involved to make it a reality. Change, such as the implementation of the FLIGHT Model, will not happen without leadership support. A manager's power is key to transformative change (Gesme & Wiseman, 2010). Nursing leaders are instrumental in creating structurally empowering workplace conditions for their employees. In this type of environment, employees feel more inclined to trust that their best interest is in mind. "Healthcare organizations should provide nursing leaders with resources that enable them to redesign nursing work environments and care processes to optimize professional nursing practice" (Erickson, Jones, & Ditomassi, 2013, p. 47). When the leaders are involved, supportive, and communicative with their employees, the planned change will be that much more successful.

When planning for change, it is important to develop and maintain a culture that promotes and rewards change. Employees must feel confident and comfortable in proposing an idea for potential change. A unit or organization that is prepared for change has a culture that looks for ways to improve and promotes ways to enhance quality, patient care, and efficiency (Gesme & Wiseman, 2010). Organizational cultures that support and welcome change are free from complacency. It is important to have members of the team who welcome change and in return are supported and rewarded for their empowerment.

Our clinical nurse who proposed the idea of the FLIGHT Model was comfortable with and felt welcomed by her leadership team to share her thoughts. If it were not for this type of culture, many creative thoughts and ideas from clinical employees would be lost. Before implementing a large change, such as redesigning a new unit council structure, ensure that your vision is clear, there is adequate leadership support, and your culture is prepared for this change.

Implementing Unit-Based Change

We recommend trialing a large change process, such as a new unit council structure, on one or two units prior to implementing it throughout the organization. Trialing on a unit may lessen fear and resistance, and it allows for learning and tweaking processes or workflows to improve any potential problems uncovered. Change is continuous and ever evolving. Small changes will continue to be made throughout the overarching change process. We trialed the FLIGHT Model for an extended period on a medical-surgical unit before spreading system-wide. This trial was successful and increased the confidence of other unit council chairs and coaches that this model would be able to work on other units as well. Additionally, the trial provided us with valuable information about the time and effort needed to implement it across the health system.

Implementing Organizational Change

When implementing a change throughout an organization, it is useful, and some say necessary, to have change agents that lead and support others and create an environment that promotes the desired change. Characteristics of great change agents that can successfully influence others include those who (Marshall & Broome, 2017, p. 49):

- Are trustworthy, reliable, honest, and credible
- Possess persuasion, negotiation, and effective listening skills
- Embody leadership through demonstration of a strong work ethic
- Are enthusiastic and show respect for individual differences
- Organize thoughts logically
- Possess strong communication skills

Because every organization is unique, it is important to remember that the change process will look and feel different for everyone and, like building a house, usually takes longer than expected. While change is constant, there are times when certain goals require fast-paced or disruptive change. Effective leaders must realize that while it is important to think about how change affects people, it is also necessary to think about how the execution of any change can make a difference in employee responses and performance (Marshall & Broome, 2017). Implementing a change organization-wide involves a larger number of people, and each person has a specific idea or assumption about how the change will affect him or her. The overall goal in this type of large organizational change is to have as many people on the same page as possible. This is when unit-level change agents and supporters come into play. Naturally there will be some resisters, but it is important to make sure everyone knows the benefits of the proposed change.

When we implemented the FLIGHT Model health-system-wide, some of our smaller units struggled to adapt to the new structure. Because the traditional model worked for them in the past, we spent significant time explaining the benefits of transitioning to the FLIGHT Model, provided support and education, and even provided at-the-elbow communication with their leaders. Most units were able to clearly understand how this new structure would improve their councils and their unit-specific outcomes.

When launching a transformative change, creating a plan is essential. "Communicate the who, what, where, why, and how of the change. Communicate the vision of what's going to happen, how individuals will be involved, what is expected from them, and why it is important" (Gesme & Wiseman, 2010,

p. 258). With a larger group of people affected by organizational change, individual needs will be different. Communication platforms will look different on each unit for their specific employees. Whether you post something in the break room, send emails, make phone calls, or discuss at employee meetings, communicating the message must be clear. Clear communication will also be a process as some employees are more involved than others. Continue to communicate the change frequently, remembering to articulate the meaning behind the change, and why and how the change affects each employee.

Adopting a Change Theory to Lay the Groundwork for Change

Change management experts agree that how change is led makes all the difference in the organization's ability to negotiate and implement the proposed change (Marshall & Broome, 2017). Because each organization is unique, identifying and implementing a change management theory that fits well with your organization is important. The FLIGHT Model is based on John Kotter's Change Theory, which is woven throughout the remainder of the book.

Change is challenging, but understanding the various stages involved in a change process allows you to anticipate actions that need to be addressed in the process. It is important to recognize and address all stages of change so that you successfully build the proper foundation to proceed and positively influence your chances of sustaining the change. By explaining the "why" behind the need for change, understanding how to gain support for your vision, empowering others, celebrating the little successes, and sustaining the energy and enthusiasm for change, you can create a lasting change that drives improvement and sustains the ongoing momentum for continual growth.

Incorporating a change theory model will help you implement a new unit council structure for your organization; it will also be beneficial in driving smaller unit-based changes. While we will illustrate the benefits of using John Kotter's Change Theory as we implemented the FLIGHT Model, there are many different change theorists that can be used. Two such theorists are William Bridges and Kurt Lewin.

William Bridges' Transition Model of Change

Bridges' Transition Model is the idea that change is situational and transition is psychological. His model focuses on the psychological transitions that take place when change occurs. *Transition* "is a three-phase process that people go through as they internalize and come to terms with the details of the new situation that the change brings about" (Bridges & Bridges, 2016, p. 3). It is important to note the emotional and internal responses that take place during change. This model is not necessarily about the change process itself, but the transition of change affecting each individual involved; it identifies the positive and negative emotions evoked through the stages of change.

His model outlines three phases:

- The ending phase
- The neutral zone
- The new beginnings

The Ending Phase

This is the first stage people enter when they are presented with an idea for change. It is the end of the current state; the letting go of what was. When an idea for change is first proposed, there may be feelings of resistance, anger, and reservation (Muir, 2017). There are likely questions of doubt and confusion as to why change needs to occur in the first place. It is important to note that change inevitably causes some kind of loss, and it is the losses that people are reacting to, not necessarily the changes (Bridges & Bridges, 2016). Leaders need to openly acknowledge the emotions that their team may be going through; otherwise, there may be a greater resistance to the change. When emotions are acknowledged, employees will know their opinions matter, and the phasing out of the old ways will run more smoothly.

The Neutral Zone

The neutral zone is the transition between the end of the current state and the new beginning. Some people may experience anxiety and hesitation about entering into a new state, but there may also be feelings of excitement or creativity as early adapters realize the potential for positive change (Bridges & Bridges, 2016). During the neutral zone, it is advantageous to embrace setbacks and encourage opportunities for innovative thinking (Bridges &

Bridges, 2016). Some people may experience discouragement and resentment, and it is important for leaders to support those hesitant about the proposed change. This phase is crucial in developing solutions and encouraging buy-in and engagement.

The New Beginnings

In the last phase of Bridges' Model, people have learned to embrace the new change leading to feelings of excitement, accomplishment, and purpose (Bridges & Bridges, 2016). Participation and collaboration increase as people conclude this final transition, but change can never be forced. Beginnings are a natural process that need encouragement and support (Bridges & Bridges, 2016). While every individual will respond differently, it is important to be patient with the final phase. The strong presence of leadership is continually valuable through every phase of Bridges' Model.

Bridges' Model can easily be utilized with the implementation of the FLIGHT Model in your organization. As the process of change occurs, there will be varying emotions about the concept of a redesigned (or new) unit council structure. Some employees may welcome it with open arms and look forward to its benefits, and others may have some doubt and denial about the need to change. It is important to acknowledge where employees are with their feelings about the proposed change. Involving them in the process will increase your opportunity for success. Figure 6.1 illustrates Bridges' Model.

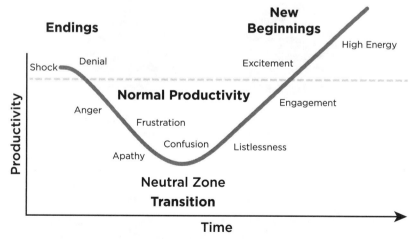

FIGURE 6.1   Bridges' Model for managing change.
(Source taken from Muir, 2017, para. 2)

Kurt Lewin's Theory of Change Model

While Bridges' Model focuses on the psychological transitions that occur during change, another theorist to consider is Kurt Lewin. Lewin's theory includes three stages of change:

- Unfreeze

- Change

- Freeze or (Refreeze)

These three stages identify the feelings of stepping outside one's comfort zone and preparing for change, or *unfreezing*. The next step is the reaction to the change and moving toward the intended direction, or the *change* step. Lastly, Lewin identifies the new normal as the *refreeze* (Connelly, 2016). Figure 6.2 is a visual depiction of Lewin's Theory of Change.

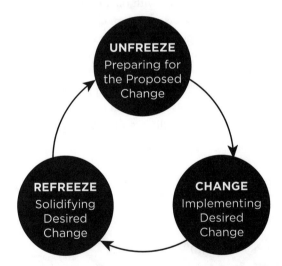

FIGURE 6.2   Kurt Lewin's Theory of Change.
(Figure created with information taken from Connelly, 2016)

Unfreeze

This stage is about getting out of a comfort zone and preparing for the proposed change. There may be feelings of anger and denial in this phase because many people are uncomfortable with change in general. Lewin created "The Force Field Analysis," which determines if the benefits of the proposed change outweigh the potential issues (Connelly, 2016). If the factors for the change outweigh the factors against the change, then the change can occur and employees are motivated to participate in the proposed change.

Change

The second phase in Lewin's three-step model is the process of implementing the desired change. This is the transition that takes place during the change process and will likely take the longest. Transition is the journey made in reaction to the change. This second stage is when people are "unfrozen" and moving toward the new change (Connelly, 2016). In this step, it is important for leaders to support the employee through the change process and to be patient with the length of time it takes to move to the next step.

Refreeze

This phase represents the new normal, once the change takes place. The proposed change has been accepted by the majority and employees are more comfortable with what has taken place. This is when the new change is solidified (Connelly, 2016). It is important to note that no change is ever complete or officially "over." It is a cycle that takes place as adaptations are made to the intended idea for change. Once a change is implemented, there will be an ongoing need for improvements or alterations.

Lewin's Theory of Change can be applied to the implementation of the FLIGHT Model by carefully assessing the three stages of change that he identifies. Before we implemented the FLIGHT Model, a work group was formed, and the appropriate team was created to prepare for the proposed change. Once the vision was created and a successful trial had occurred, the desired change was implemented across all units. In the final stage, the proposed change was solidified.

Kotter's Theory of Change and Its Use in the FLIGHT Model

John Kotter is the change theorist we used in the development of the FLIGHT Model. His Theory of Change includes eight steps of transformational change and is widely used throughout various industries and organizations. Kotter's Change Process clearly outlines eight stages of planned change. In this process, he explains that the first four steps "help defrost a hardened status quo...

Phases five to seven then introduce many new practices. The last stage grounds the changes in the corporate culture and helps make them stick" (Kotter, 2012, p. 24). It is important to create a climate for change and engage employees, implement the change, and sustain the change. It is crucial to not skip steps through the transformation process because the foundation needs to be strong and durable for a system to tolerate the change and ultimately to sustain the new way of working. Figure 6.3 is a visual depiction of Kotter's Theory of Change.

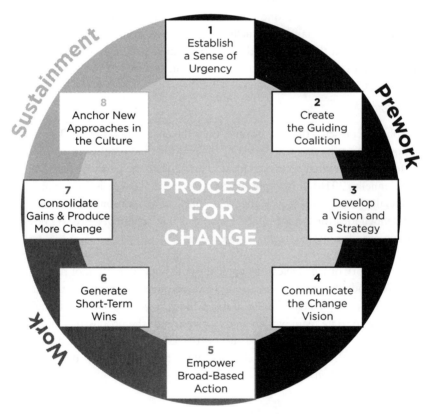

FIGURE 6.3   Kotter's Theory—8-step process for leading change.
(Adapted from Kotter, Inc., 2018)

As Kotter expresses in his work, it is imperative that every step is taken and completed before moving on to the next stage. If a change agent jumps from establishing a sense of urgency to communicating the change vision, that agent will immediately lose any potential success because the adequate team was not created, and the strategy was lost. Change takes time, as will each of the steps to create successful change.

Through application of Kotter's Theory of Change, the eight steps are defined and applied using case studies. There are four characteristics repeated through the case studies; these are the pillars of the FLIGHT Model as illustrated in Chapter 3, Figure 3.2. The pillars include: engagement of the interprofessional team, leadership support, alignment with organization goals, and adequate communication.

Kotter Step 1: Establish a Sense of Urgency

> 1
> Establish a Sense of Urgency

Establishing a sense of urgency is the first step of the change process. With the pace of change in healthcare and multiple competing priorities, a sense of urgency is key in bringing the necessary attention to the problem at hand and the need to provide solutions that involve changing practice or beliefs. Establishing a sense of urgency helps others to see the importance of the idea and why it should even be considered. Establishing urgency often involves sharing the "why" behind the need for change. It allows leaders and peers to "feel" the necessity of the change and to understand why it must happen now, rather than down the road. Having leaders and peers understand the importance of "why now?" is crucial in setting the stage for the next step—creating a guiding coalition.

CASE STUDY: Establishing a Sense of Urgency

Registered nurses on a specialty medical stroke unit receive annual stroke specialty training to properly care for this unique population of patients. In a recent employee meeting, nursing leadership shared with all team members that a new position had been hired to build the neuroscience service line, including increasing the number of stroke patients that would be cared for on this unit. A nursing aide approached the unit leader expressing a concern that there was not adequate education for the nursing assistants who worked on this unit regarding their part in caring for the stroke patients and requested that there be role-specific stroke education for nursing assistants. The nursing assistant elaborated to the leader that with an increase in stroke patients, it was imperative that this education happen sooner rather than later and requested courses begin within one month. The leader valued the input from the team member and understood the CNA's sense of urgency to start planning the training. The CNA's urgency to have stroke training for the nursing assistant team helped other team members to have that same sense of urgency and desire to organize in-services. A clinical RN on the team collaborated with an interprofessional group of physical, occupational, and speech therapists to develop a series of in-services for the nursing aides on the floor. This collaborative series of in-services provided audience-appropriate education on the identification and pathophysiology of stroke, safe ways to improve the patient's activities of daily living, and their role in the care of this vulnerable population. The therapists also discussed ways to be mindful of the employee's own personal safety while mobilizing hemispheric patients to avoid employee injury. The result was an increase in teamwork, employee satisfaction, and improved care and safety measures for this patient population and the care team. Because the CNA shared his idea with a sense of urgency, he was able to engage others to see the value of the request and gain support of the CNA's role as a vital part of the care team.

Kotter Step 2: Create the Guiding Coalition

In the stage of forming a powerful guiding coalition, the project team is assembled. This team feels the urgency and necessity for change and works together to plan and lead the identified change. This stage requires strong team-building, trust, and collaboration. Four characteristics essential to effective guiding coalitions are (Kotter, 2012):

- Position power
- Expertise
- Credibility
- Leadership

These characteristics generate the understanding that all opinions are valid for consideration and all members are respected and are on an equal playing field. It is necessary to find the right people, create trust, and develop a common goal. Having the right team together supports the collaboration needed for the next stage—developing a vision and a strategy.

CASE STUDY: Forming a Powerful Guiding Coalition

A medical unit cared for an average of 350 patients each month, yet the number of patient satisfaction survey responses averaged only nine responses per month. The clinical nurses on this unit wondered about the other 341 patients who experienced care on their unit.

Two nurses on the unit identified an area for improvement: increasing the number of patient survey responses to obtain more information on overall patient satisfaction. These nurses were informal leaders on their unit and added credibility to the change project.

As they began their work, they quickly realized they lacked knowledge on the patient satisfaction survey process. They formed a work group that included unit leadership, the coordinator of patient satisfaction, and a few employees who had been former patients. The two nurses became the designated project leaders. Though there were organizational leaders in the group, the project was employee-driven and presented an opportunity to develop employees as leaders.

The group met, and each member provided valuable contributions to the project. The coordinator of patient satisfaction provided information on the patient survey process and appropriate ways to solicit survey participation. She was the team member with expertise and a person with the appropriate position power. The director provided the leadership role that was necessary to ensure any changes that were undertaken could be operationalized on the unit. This director would also facilitate collaboration with necessary experts, derail road blocks, and provide support as needed. Although in a leadership role, the director was NOT the lead of this group. The employees who were former patients understood their employee role but were also able to provide insight regarding the patient's perspective (more levels of expertise). All members of the project group worked together as a cohesive team—understanding each other's roles, the valuable contributions each person could offer, and trusting in the collaborative and professional process they were engaged in.

This group had found the right people, created trust, and developed a common goal of increasing patient survey response rates. Without both leadership and group team support, the team leaders would not have been successful in developing a plan or seen their power make a difference. This guiding coalition was imperative to empowerment for change. Because there was a guiding coalition in place, the third phase of change could be tackled—developing a vision and a strategy to address survey response numbers.

Kotter Step 3: Develop a Vision and a Strategy

After forming the guiding coalition, or project team, it is important to develop a vision and a strategy for the group to achieve the proposed change. According to Kotter (2012), creating a vision helps to direct the efforts and serves three purposes:

- The vision clarifies the general direction for change.

- The vision motivates people to take action in an aligned direction.

- The vison helps coordinate the actions of different people in an efficient manner.

In this third step, it is important to clarify the benefits of the future change and how the team can aid in turning the idea into reality. Once a vision and strategy are developed, the map for change is outlined. Having this vision defined with a strategy in mind allows the process to move to the next stage—communicating the change vision to others.

CASE STUDY: Developing a Vision and a Strategy

Several nurses and CNAs formed a group to look at increasing patient satisfaction scores and improving patient safety through hourly rounding. The project lead was a clinical nurse with a passion for patient satisfaction and a zeal to keep patients safe by reducing falls.

Through the project lead's direction, the group elected to implement strategies that would both increase patient satisfaction scores related to responsiveness and reduce patient falls. To accomplish both objectives (the entire vision), the strategy they chose was purposeful hourly rounding.

Because hourly rounding had been trialed in the past and was not successful, the team (the guiding coalition) wanted to create a plan for sustained change. To help with project scope and direction, they began their work by mapping out a project board with milestones and a timeline to outline the project's general direction. The project board and timeline helped to motivate team members because they now knew the direction and focus of the project.

With multiple interprofessional employees on the committee, mapping out project tasks on a timeline helped to define and distribute the project workload among the group. This reduced the chances of duplicating work and allowed a more efficient process for project development and completion.

Once the vision and strategy were clear to the team, they were able to begin work developing the unit's hourly rounding plan. The goal was to increase patient satisfaction, lower the amount of call lights, and decrease falls through hourly rounding by preemptively addressing patients' needs.

Because the group had formed their vision and developed a plan, they were ready to enter the next stage of the change process—communicating the change vision to their peers to gain their support for, and even participation in, the planned process change.

| 4 |
| Communicate |
| the Change |
| Vision |

Kotter Step 4: Communicate the Change Vision

A shared sense of an ideal future can help motivate and coordinate actions into transformations. Failing to effectively communicate the proposed vision will, without a doubt, hinder the change process. Keeping the message simple and clear is required for effective vision communication. The two-minute elevator speech is a way to describe a message that is simple and clear, where the listener understands the intended message or vision. It may also be helpful to use metaphor, analogy, and examples to illustrate the vision (Kotter, 2012). When the project team uses examples to illustrate the message, the listener is better able to understand the vision. This understanding allows an opportunity for listener input into the change vision and leads to their participation in the change action. By engaging and informing others of the vision and planned strategy, the project team has a strong foundation to move into the fifth stage of change—empowering broad-based action.

CASE STUDY: Communicating the Change Vision

On a busy medical renal unit, missing breakfast became a common concern voiced by several patients receiving hemodialysis, due to the delivery time. The unit supervisor/charge nurse and the director of nutritional services met to identify the root cause of this complaint. They developed a plan for an improvement process that allowed for all hemodialysis patients with a diet order to automatically receive early breakfast trays.

This early tray process, however, would create a change in workflow. The night shift (instead of the day shift) would now be responsible to receive and serve the breakfast trays along with any necessary meal medications. This would occur at the end of their shift during a very busy time. The project team recognized that this would affect the night shift workflow and understood that early communication of the process change would be imperative for all employees to share the ideal future vision.

This early meal change was widely communicated by unit leadership to the employees through several emails and unit shift huddle announcements. They detailed the change and the workflow expectation as well as the "why" behind the change. All employees understood the background to the vision and embraced a shared sense of the ideal future to support their patients' nutrition and satisfaction. Because the need for change was thoroughly communicated, employees on both shifts collaborated on ways to incorporate the new workflow and were able to address a patient satisfaction concern.

By addressing this four-hour delay in dialysis patients receiving breakfast, individual hemodialysis patient satisfaction concerns were addressed, and there were minimal subsequent patient complaints about delayed meals.

Communicating the change vision to all affected parties is essential to the next stage of change management—encouraging broader participation and action.

Establishing a sense of urgency, forming a guiding coalition, developing a vision and a strategy, and communicating the vision strategy are the first four steps of Kotter's eight-step change process. We advise you not to skip any steps because this is the foundational work that supports future steps. These steps ensure the goal is clear to all and that all team members affected by the change have a better understanding and can support the vision. When employees understand the meaning behind a process and can explain it to another employee member, buy-in, understanding, and support will naturally occur. Frequently, the project lead and selected team members understand the vision well in advance of others. It is important to remember to go through the first four steps adequately with the rest of the team to engage others' buy-in and support to create success. You must start where the team is—and build from that. The first four stages of change are predicated on building support for the change. The next three steps are the active working stages of change.

5 Empower Broad-Based Action

Kotter Step 5: Empower Broad-Based Action

When implementing change, it is beneficial to encourage those who seek positive change and to anticipate some risk taking. In this stage, empowering broad-based action involves investing in employees and promoting leadership development. It is important for leaders to encourage employees to look outside the box for innovative change, as well as support their findings with evidence-based research. This empowerment provides an energy and involvement that supports change. When a group feels empowered to act, it generates an enthusiasm that encourages action. This is the beginning of the active working stages of change. When this stage is in motion, it is important to think about the next stage of change—generating short-term wins.

CASE STUDY: Empowering Broad-Based Action

Reducing turnaround time (TAT), or door to admission time for patients from the emergency department (ED) to the inpatient setting, was an opportunity for improvement because current times were not meeting benchmarks. Current literature and best-practice evidence improved patient outcomes by reducing the patient wait time spent in the ED. An ED TAT task force was developed to evaluate current processes and workflow barriers. Members of the task force included nursing leadership, clinical bedside nurses, nursing assistants from the ED and various inpatient departments, nurse educators, physicians, and transport employees.

The group spent three full days evaluating each step in the process from the time there was a decision to admit to the moment the patient arrived on the inpatient unit for admission. In-depth drill downs on workflow evaluated the number of attempts employees tried to communicate a hand-off report between the ED and the inpatient unit.

The group brainstormed many different variables (interruptions and barriers) and created processes utilizing the electronic medical record to help connect the ED communication to the inpatient nurse, as well as streamline the transportation process to the inpatient bed. Pilot trials were done with a few units to test the new process, and adjustments were done to make it as beneficial as possible to all parties involved. After the pilot trials were successful, the initiative was launched throughout the organization.

By involving widespread employee input of those closest to the problem, the organization empowered a broad-based action plan. This broad-based group was able to offer multiple workflow perspectives and identify a robust range of ideas for improving the process. They were able to trial their plan, evaluate, and adjust to actively work on decreasing the ED TAT and improve their patient outcomes.

6
Generate
Short-Term
Wins

Kotter Step 6: Generate Short-Term Wins

The next working stage of leading change is generating short-term wins. Recognition and celebration of small wins is important during the larger process of change. Recognizing the short-term wins rewards your change agents with a pat on the back, building morale and motivation. Short-term wins help fine-tune the vision and strategies, build momentum, and provide evidence that short-term sacrifices are worth the effort. Kotter shares that "as a general rule, the more cynics and resisters, the more important are short-term wins" (Kotter, 2012, p. 127). Short-term wins sustain the development of the change project. As recognition of these short-term successes continues along the project pathway, the next stage of change evolves—consolidating gains and producing more change.

CASE STUDY: Generate Short-Term Wins

A team of nurses and nursing assistants formed a group to create interpreter cards in five different languages. The organization had a two-page card of images and basic words, but only in English. Employees realized it would be beneficial to support individualized patient care by creating these types of cards in multiple languages. This would allow employees to easily communicate basic needs with patients who speak a different language. The communication picture cards were expanded to five pages in one language to help meet patients' basic activity of daily living and comfort needs. The language card set was trialed on the unit. Upon experiencing the short-term win of improved patient communication for basic care needs in the first language, the language cards were then developed in additional languages. The employees who created the change were recognized and rewarded. This positive reinforcement helped to build morale and boost a sense of pride in the employees and unit. The language cards were then shared with other patient care areas of the organization. A project that started as an idea generating from a workflow barrier evolved into an organizational benefit that was sustainable by acknowledging the short-term wins along the way.

| 7 |
| Consolidate |
| Gains & Produce |
| More Change |

Kotter Step 7: Consolidate Gains and Produce More Change

Having acknowledged the short-term wins during project development, the change process continues into the next working phase of consolidating gains and producing more change. When there are multiple teams working toward a common goal or vision, they may be able to help each other anticipate conflicts, prioritize plans, and commit for the overall good of the organization. In this stage, there is more change occurring, more help, and an increase in project management from the employees (Kotter, 2012). As more employees participate in the new change, support becomes widespread, and this leads to the final stage of the change process—anchor the new approach in the culture.

CASE STUDY: Consolidating Gains and Producing More Change

A unit had an idea to develop a workflow project around standardizing a location for gait belts. A nurse and physical therapist worked together to decide a standard location in the patient rooms for placing all gait belts on a hook by the door. This would enable everyone to know where to look, while saving time and frustration spent searching the patient room for the gait belt or retrieving another belt to replace the "lost" belt. A standard location also reduced costs associated with multiple gait belts piling up in the patient room.

A second unit adopted the idea after hearing about it at a leadership sharing venue. The leaders brought the idea back to their respective unit and shared it with the employees. The second unit then developed a workflow project to standardize a mobility kit by packaging together the gait belt and patient non-skid slippers to grab and go from the supply room to facilitate employee workflow and support patient safety.

Using the same workflow improvement approach and brainstorming together, additional change was created and shared. By sharing the gain of a standardized gait belt location in the patient room, a second unit was motivated to focus on patient mobility and to continue to streamline workflow by developing a mobility kit. Because gains were consolidated and additional change was produced, the team could then proceed to the final stage of the change process—anchoring new approaches in the culture.

| 8 |
| Anchor New Approaches in the Culture |

Kotter Step 8: Anchor New Approaches in the Culture

Anchoring the new change into the culture is the last step in the change process; the "making it stick" part. Cultural change takes time, yet most people want to make sure a new approach will work before completely committing time and resources. Some projects that have been implemented using the FLIGHT Model have taken longer to develop than others. One reason may be the time it takes to change expectations of employees, some of whom may be resistant to change. By working to improve the communication between employees and identifying the responsibilities of each team member, an improved culture can take place. During this final phase of the change process, the new process becomes ingrained in the culture and can be sustained as it replaces the old.

CASE STUDY: Anchoring New Approaches in the Culture

An organization had a hospital-wide goal to improve the culture of safety at every level. An initiative that was implemented was the monitoring or auditing of hand hygiene (whether it was completed or not) and peer coaching for those who were witnessed as non-compliant. The challenge in performing this coaching was that not every employee had the confidence to approach a perceived higher-ranking team member. Education and leadership support were provided to all employees, allowing everyone permission and empowerment to approach anyone at any level of the organization to comment if they noticed a lack of hand hygiene. This took quite some time to get used to because some employees felt they were being disrespectful.

This practice of coaching was a huge culture change, and it took time to put into practice. Eventually every employee was held accountable for their actions to increase safety for each other and the patients they cared for. With this culture change, hand hygiene has been consistently sustained at an improved level. Team members share camaraderie proudly for finding opportunities to offer kudos for hand hygiene done well. By anchoring the hand hygiene expectations into daily practice, the number of healthcare-acquired infections has been reduced at the organization and a fundamental culture of safety has been anchored within the organization. Anchoring the desired behavior and tying it to real patient outcomes helps to ensure the practice can and will be sustained.

Putting It All Together: Reducing Hospital-Acquired Pressure Injuries (HAPIs) Using the FLIGHT Model

Analysis of Current State

A healthcare organization wanted to reduce the number of hospital-acquired pressure injuries (HAPIs) it was experiencing. The nursing division was searching for best practice interventions shared by other facilities. Many of the evidence-based best practices had already been implemented, but the organization still grappled with the question, "What can we do that will truly make a difference and reduce the occurrence of HAPIs?"

An observant clinical nurse, Tina, noted that some of the HAPIs were not truly hospital-acquired. Occasionally, when a nurse found a pressure injury, the patient or family would comment that it was not a new injury, but rather something they were aware of prior to admission. Because the nurses did not identify the pressure injury within the required time from admission, it was considered hospital-acquired due to nationally established criteria. Tina understood that thorough skin assessments were not a priority for all employees despite the untoward outcomes for the patient and the negative reimbursement implications.

Tina was aware that an organization located in their regional area had experienced no HAPIs in the prior year, so she began to ask herself some questions:

- What did this organization do differently?
- What specific actions could she do to champion and lead efforts to decrease HAPIs in her organization?

Some of the similarities included various pressure prevention surfaces, routine repositioning of patients, skin assessment/intervention scoring rubric, appropriate nutritional support, transfer devices to reduce shearing risk, skincare products to add moisture protection from incontinence, foam dressings to protect skin pressure areas, a dedicated skin and wound team plus additional wound resource nurses on each unit, as well as ongoing employee training. She did note one practice difference, however. The organization that had no HAPIs utilized a two-clinical-nurse skin assessment upon admission to the inpatient setting. This assessment was done within a specified time frame and included a full-body skin assessment.

1
Establish a Sense of Urgency

Kotter Step 1: Establish a Sense of Urgency

Tina approached her unit leadership team with her idea of implementing this practice change but anticipated for the work group to establish the specific time frames for skin assessments. The leadership team verified the need to address HAPI reduction because their unit-specific data indicated the occurrences of HAPI were higher than the year prior and climbing (organizational alignment).

The manager's interest was piqued, and he was open to evaluating the evidence Tina shared about the practice at another facility. The manager recommended Tina use the FLIGHT Model for the unit council professional governance process to develop her idea and provided a copy of the FLIGHT Project Toolkit to help her get started. The manager and Tina then met with the unit council chair to share the project idea. The manager, council chair, and Tina reviewed the toolkit together to support the clinical nurse's understanding of the FLIGHT toolkit and process.

In the toolkit, the first item necessary to complete is the FLIGHT SBAR (see Appendix B). The SBAR tool is a format that is familiar to the clinical nurse, easily understood, and easy to complete. Following are highlights of this SBAR:

SBAR: HAPI Incidence Rates

- **Situation:** High incidence of HAPIs in current organization and specifically on this unit

- **Background:** Another organization has experienced no HAPIs for the prior year.

- **Assessment:** Thorough skin assessments are not routinely a priority for all employees. Despite the organizational campus, skin prevention practices at all facilities were identical or very similar. No process or expectation currently exists for two-nurse skin assessments upon admission.

- **Recommendation:** Trial a program to provide an increased collegial focus on skin assessments.

HAPI Incidence Reduction: A Quality Improvement Project

Tina quickly completed the FLIGHT SBAR. To support the sense of urgency to start working on the project, she included the unit's Performance Improvement Dashboard report comparing the current and previous years' HAPI numbers reported to the national database, NDNQI. The HAPI incidence numbers were increasing, and the urgency to address the issue was apparent. It was clear that a change was needed for better patient outcomes.

Kotter Step 2: Create the Guiding Coalition

The clinical nurse, unit council chair, and the unit leadership team met to discuss the SBAR and strategize the best way to implement the needed change. Based on data showing incidence rates, the team decided to trial the project and interventions on the two inpatient units that were experiencing the highest number of HAPI occurrences. The units chosen included a progressive care unit and a medical-surgical unit.

The team members decided they needed to create a group of clinical nurses and leaders from both units to plan and implement the project. They invited the leadership teams and the wound resource clinical nurses from both units to a planning meeting, along with the clinical nurse educator and an IT nurse analyst. The guiding coalition was assembled.

The clinical nurse who submitted the HAPI incidence reduction project idea became the project lead. The leadership team was included at the start of the project, but the unit council coach and chair agreed their presence at ongoing project meetings was no longer necessary. While their presence at the meetings was not necessary, both the coach and the chair were readily available to support the project lead if or when she needed.

The unit council chair also shared with Tina the established monthly project reporting process, which includes the Reporting Tool and the Time Tracking Log (see Appendix C and Appendix D).

This report helps the unit council chair track project time for overall unit council budgeted hours on the Unit Council Budget Log (see Appendix E). This reporting process also allowed the unit council chair to consolidate communications into a monthly Unit Council Newsletter so all unit employees receive updates on ongoing unit projects.

Kotter Step 3: Develop a Vision and a Strategy

At the initial meeting, the clinical nurse Tina, who was now the project lead, shared her FLIGHT SBAR and her ideas for the project with the newly formed work group. The work group was acutely aware of the urgent need for change and improvement in this important clinical outcome. They were eager to develop the vision and a strategy to achieve a positive outcome.

The name for the project was "4 Eyes in 4 Hours." The work group agreed that this name clearly described the initiative and made the two-nurse skin assessment task achievable for clinical employees to incorporate into their workflow. The established process that was developed required two clinical nurses performing the skin assessment together within four hours of patient arrival. The goal of this project was to increase the number of appropriate skin interventions being implemented and decrease the time from assessment to intervention deployment.

After pinning down the timeline, the group brainstormed the best way to develop an action plan (see Appendix F). They developed a timeline for planned employee education and secured a launch date of the pilot program. They also developed an audit tool for the charge nurses to help monitor shift just-in-time compliance and support employee awareness of proper skin assessments with the new 4 Eyes in 4 Hours process.

The group determined that charge nurse audits of the 4 Eyes in 4 Hours documentation would continue until the unit met a sustained 90% documentation compliance for 60 days. Upon meeting this goal, the audits were planned to be reduced to random spot checks with follow-up to employees as necessary. A friendly competition developed between the two trial units to see who could achieve the documentation goal first. The employees were beginning to envision the future as a reality.

Kotter Step 4: Communicate the Change Vision

4 Eyes in 4 Hours

The two units shared a sense of the ideal state they wanted to achieve. After developing the vision and strategy, the group knew it was time to formally communicate the proposed 4 Eyes in 4 Hours project to the employees of both pilot units and launch the employee education. The project action plan was updated, and the clinical employees worked with the clinical nurse educator to develop an education plan. The plan included poster boards with information regarding the number of HAPIs the units had recently experienced—which conveyed a sense of urgency to the employees. The poster boards explained the "why" behind the initiatives of:

- Focus on improving skin assessments done upon admission/arrival to the unit.

- Immediately identify pressure injuries that existed prior to admission.

- Identify potential pressure areas at risk, and implement skin interventions in a timely manner.

- Reduce the overall number of HAPI occurrences.

By educating the "why" behind the initiative, employees had a clearer understanding of the planned project and could support the change in their workflow.

The team set a goal of widespread unit communication to garner employee acceptance of the vision and strategy. The communication centered on the proposed plan of accomplishing a two-clinical-nurse skin assessment with appropriate documentation within four hours of patient arrival to the unit. The clinical nurses on the project team and the unit leadership shared the education at shift huddles and provided one-on-one employee education as necessary to communicate the change vision and engage other employees. By engaging and educating these key stakeholders about the vision, the project team completed the pre-work stages of change and were ready for the active work of implementing the change.

5
Empower Broad-Based Action

Kotter Step 5: Empower Broad-Based Action

Enough time was planned for unit communications prior to the project launch date. This helped to ensure a broad-based awareness of the plan and allowed time for questions to be answered about the process and the new documentation co-sign plan. Employees understood the rationale for the process. Some of the project team members started informally performing the two-clinical-nurse 4 Eyes assessments to further identify potential barriers for the process. While these nurses were doing their informal 4 Eyes assessments, they began to involve nonproject team members as well. They engaged both the clinical nurses on the unit as well as the nursing assistants, which allowed further educational opportunities and promoted a broad employee engagement in the initiative. These team members felt empowered to achieve this change. Their enthusiasm encouraged action from others and illustrated to the team readiness to implement fully and put the vision into action.

6
Generate Short-Term Wins

Kotter Step 6: Generate Short-Term Wins

The employee education communication had been completed and the IT nurse analyst had finished the electronic medical record update—two items to close out on the project action plan.

The project launch date arrived, and the pilot units were eager and willing to trial the new 4 Eyes in 4 Hours process. The charge nurses had the audit sheets and were ready to start their chart reviews and offer support and reminders to employees on this new initiative.

The project team evaluated the audit sheets weekly and crunched the numbers, eagerly anticipating the day when the units would meet 90% chart audit documentation compliance of 4 Eyes in 4 Hours. Each unit posted its audit results and recruited its employees into a friendly competition with peers on the other pilot unit. Who would make it to the 90% compliance first? The project team was aware that it might take a few months to consistently reach the 90% goal. By posting the weekly audit results, it allowed an opportunity to create a visible reminder of the initiative. As compliance improved, the units were able to celebrate their short-term wins on a weekly basis. Those individual employees who were performing exceptionally well with their compliance were also recognized during daily huddles. These types of celebrations sustained the development of the change project and encouraged other members of the unit to participate and support the momentum as well.

| 7 |
| Consolidate Gains & Produce More Change |

Kotter Step 7: Consolidate Gains and Produce More Change

Employees provided feedback to the project team. The focus on skin assessments and interventions generated more thoughts on what could be done to support the patient's skin and reduce pressure ulcers. Support for the project was growing among the two units. The suggestion was made by employees to broaden the 4 Eyes practice to include not only new patients arriving to the unit but also those current patients who were off the unit for over two hours for a procedure. Employees observed that patients lying on various surfaces, such as procedure tables or gurneys, for an extended length of time often returned with reddened pressure areas.

The employees were also concerned about high-skin-risk patients as determined by a daily skin risk assessment score, which prompted the suggestion to broaden the 4 Eyes practice to include a skin assessment on any patient that scored as high-skin-risk on the daily assessment (or those patients deemed at higher risk for skin breakdown due to their co-morbidities).

The addition of these two elements meant more work for the clinical employees. However, this additional workflow was embraced because the employees felt empowered and realized their nursing care made a difference.

The charge nurse audit sheets were updated to reflect the additional assessments. Support for 4 Eyes in 4 Hours had become widespread among the two units. After six months, the employees were seeing a decrease in the number of reported HAPIs. They also reported being more confident in their skin assessment skills. By partnering for the skin assessments, they could easily collaborate on a concerning skin finding and determine an appropriate plan of care.

| 8 |
| Anchor New Approaches in the Culture |

Kotter Step 8: Anchor New Approaches in the Culture

The project team was eager to share its success with other units in the organization. One of the trial units experienced a 24% reduction in reportable HAPIs after the first year of implementation. The project leader presented the project and the improved outcomes to the nursing division's leadership team. This venue included 60 nurse leaders from adult inpatient services. The positive outcomes were well received, and the nurse leaders of other units asked if it was possible to implement this initiative hospital-wide.

The project leader updated her project action plan to include a rollout plan to other adult inpatient units. The team created educational binders for the on-boarding units to explain the background, the 4 Eyes in 4 Hours process, and the charge nurse audit tool. These were shared among the division along with a start date for everyone to begin. The pilot units were excited to see their project spreading. The two pilot units were available to provide support and answer questions as the rest of the division adopted the practice into their settings. The trial units shared their statistical successes, which motivated the on-boarding units to become engaged quickly. After the first year of implementation, the organization saw an overall reduction in reportable HAPIs, including a further 60% reduction on the original trial unit. The clinical employees and leadership team were committed to achieving their goal. Because of this dedication and commitment, the 4 Eyes in 4 Hours process became ingrained in the culture and has proven to be sustainable.

The Power of the FLIGHT Model

The HAPI reduction unit council project is a clear example of how the FLIGHT Model, once implemented, can lead to successful projects, both large and small. An engaged clinical nurse felt empowered to propose an idea for change that was appropriately aligned with organizational goals, was supported by leadership, and included a clearly communicated vision.

Additionally, the case studies provided illustrate the pathways defined by John Kotter to successfully implement change. Selecting a change theorist prior to implementing change is imperative in recognizing different phases of change and how they relate to the needs of your organization. We find Kotter's theory best guides us in our ever-changing healthcare environment today. With this solid foundation in place, we can now move on to the practical tools and training necessary to implement the FLIGHT Model.

References

Bridges, W., & Bridges, S. (2016). *Managing transitions: Making the most of change* (4th ed.). Boston, MA: Da Capo Lifelong Books.

Connelly, M. (2016, November 15). *The Kurt Lewin change management model.* Retrieved from https://www.change-management-coach.com/kurt_lewin.html

Erickson, J. I., Jones, D. A., & Ditomassi, M. (2013). *Fostering nurse-led care: Professional practice for the bedside leader from Massachusetts General Hospital.* Indianapolis, IN: Sigma Theta Tau International.

Gesme, D., & Wiseman, M. (2010). How to implement change in practice. *Journal of Oncology Practice, 6*(5), 257–259. http://doi.org/10.1200/JOP.000089

Kotter, Inc. (2018). *8 steps to accelerate change.* Retrieved from https://www.kotterinc.com/8-steps-process-for-leading-change/

Kotter, J. P. (2012). *Leading change.* Boston, MA: *Harvard Business Review.*

Marshall, E. S., & Broome, M. (2017). *Transformational leadership in nursing: From expert clinician to influential leader.* New York, NY: Springer Publishing Company.

Muir, R., Esq. (2017, October 25). Successfully making changes. *Law People Blog.com.* Retrieved from https://www.lawpeopleblog.com/2017/10/successfully-making-changes

"A dream doesn't become reality through magic; it takes sweat, determination, and hard work."

–Colin Powell

7

GETTING THE FLIGHT MODEL OFF THE GROUND: TOOLS AND TRAINING

- Understand the importance of having standardized tools
- Identify how to use the tools throughout various phases of a project

Historically, unit councils faced many challenges. Although the council members represented their unit and had visions of supporting ideas and implementing change to improve outcomes, most ideas came from noncouncil members' complaints. These complaints were often unloaded on the unit council with the unrealistic expectation that the council would solve the problems and therefore improve employee satisfaction, frustrations with the work environment, patient satisfaction, and clinical outcomes. Additionally, formal leaders did not understand the purpose of the unit council and would assign council members work to do, like review and edit policies or audit charts for a purpose outside of the unit council's focus. In other situations, the unit councils were asked by peers to do things they did not have authority to do, like improve staffing by hiring more clinical employees or change practice by purchasing a piece of equipment without considering budget or policies and procedures. This historical approach created feelings of disappointment and resentment. Council members felt like they were set up to fail. In order to be successful, they felt a need to put in time and work above and beyond what felt realistic. Ultimately, unit council members felt they were letting their peers down because they were not able to implement their unit's desired changes. At the same time, noncouncil members experienced frustration because they did not feel heard by their council or that their idea was supported, and they lost faith in the governance structure.

The FLIGHT Model can help solve some of these historical challenges by making it easier for any employee to create or be involved in a change. The FLIGHT Model supports employees stepping forward to engage and seek out opportunities to make a difference. Ideas or frustrations that may have historically been off-loaded onto a unit council are now encouraged to be owned by all. One of the most revolutionary shifts in the FLIGHT Model is the removal of unit council meetings. With the FLIGHT Model, there are tools and processes that are accessible to all. These clear pathways give each employee the opportunity to make a difference, experience personal growth, and feel empowered to turn a pain point or a frustration into a positive outcome for patients, families, and colleagues.

FLIGHT Simulator: Tools and Training

If your unit council is struggling to get projects off the ground or to increase employee engagement, the FLIGHT Model and its tools can help move innovative ideas forward by:

- Using standardized tools and processes for communicating an idea and creating a project plan
- Clarifying roles and responsibilities so all members understand their role and how they can contribute to the success of the project
- Shifting "meeting time" budget to "project" budget so employees are paid for their project work
- Increasing exposure and spread of unit projects through project presentation opportunities

The FLIGHT Model Toolkit

The FLIGHT Model Solutions/Toolkit includes the following:

- Letter of support from CNO
- Budget
- Unit project pathway
- FLIGHT Tool 1: SBAR to communicate the idea for change
- FLIGHT Tool 2: Reporting tool to communicate progress and barriers
- FLIGHT Tool 3: Time tracking log for project members to track their hours
- FLIGHT Tool 4: Budget log
- FLIGHT Tool 5: Project action plan to outline the actions, the owner of the action, and the timing of the action
- Roles and responsibilities
- Support and resources

Leadership Letter of Support

The first page of the toolkit is a letter of support from the CNO. Showing leadership and organizational support of the model is essential before the tools are explored and the process mapped out. Having a letter from the CNO (or another key leader at the executive level) sends a clear message that leadership supports professional governance and the work of the clinical teams. According to Joseph and Bogue (2018), "The primary mechanism for influencing workplace culture is leadership. This mechanism includes the actions and behaviors of leaders, what gets rewarded or discouraged by the leaders, and where leaders allocate resources" (p. 395). Making the shift from a more traditional unit council structure, with a set number of council members who meet regularly to accomplish their work, to a nontraditional approach, like the FLIGHT Model, can be uncomfortable for many. It is during these times that leadership at all levels of the organization is looked to for guidance and support.

Budget

In conjunction with the CNO letter of support, it is important to have an organized and equitable budget. The budget should clearly allocate resources to support project work and prevent disparity across units. Budgeting for indirect nursing time associated with professional governance activities (council meetings, project work, and professional development) can be a challenge for leadership (Saladino & Gosselin, 2014). With the FLIGHT Model, there is no longer a need to have unit council meetings. The resources allocated to support council meetings are now shifted to support project work. This shift is often well received by clinical employees who historically experience frustration with meetings.

Many council chairs, with the traditional unit council structure, experienced difficulty running a successful meeting. Unit council meetings often pulled clinical nurses out of the staffing mix and created a tension between those on the council and those not on the council. If a unit council meeting was held during a time where staffing was short, members were often pulled out of the meeting to provide patient care. Other times, meetings were held on the unit to help make it easier for clinical nurses to attend. This often led to a meeting full of distractions: phones ringing, clinical nurses exiting and entering the meeting to check on a patient or tend to a priority, and other interruptions. Because staffing demands take precedence over council meetings, unit council chairs were often challenged with running a productive and efficient meeting.

FLIGHT Simulator: Meeting Challenges and Budgetary Impact

Have you considered the expense of unit council meetings? Are you getting the most out of your council meetings? Could there be a better way?

- If a unit council has eight members and meets 10 times/year for two hours, 160 hours of paid time is set aside for meetings.
- If the average salary of the meeting participant is $50/hour, $8,000 a year is spent on meeting time.
- Unit council meetings can have multiple interruptions, poor attendance, and feel unproductive.
- Would it be more beneficial to shift budgeted time from meetings to projects?

The FLIGHT Model budget was built to support project work for the project lead and project team members. Additional time was allotted for the chair to work with the coach to support the project leads and project team members.

The budget seen in Figure 7.1 is for acute care inpatient units, emergency departments, and surgical areas to support three concurrent projects per unit. Allocations are adjusted according to unit size to allow appropriate support for smaller teams. Ideally, there is little disparity across the organization, and each unit should feel it has a budget that is representative of its needs.

	Monthly Hours	Yearly Hours
Chair	6	72
Project Leads (4 hours x 3 potential leads)	12	144
Project members (3 hours x 6 members – or 2 members/project)	18	216
Total	36	432

FIGURE 7.1   FLIGHT Model budget for unit council projects.

Budget assumptions:

- Applies to inpatient units, emergency departments, and surgical areas.
- One chair
- Three project leads—one for each focus area:
    - Employee satisfaction
    - Quality outcomes
    - Patient satisfaction
- Two employee team members for each project lead and focus area.
- Smaller departments (depending on executive level approval for area) may have up to eight hours for project work.
- Chairs will maintain accurate log and monitoring of hours for each project and project lead.
- Unit council chair meeting held every other month would come from a central budget dedicated to Magnet redesignation costs.
- Any report or meetings for project leads and chairs would come out of the Magnet budget.
- Council project supplies and funds needed for rewarding project completion, employee recognition, and so on would come from unit budgets.

Project Pathway

Our new unit council model encourages widespread participation and an understanding that ideas of any scope and scale can be put into action. Our intent was to create a model that would fit any lifestyle, work schedule, and level of experience as well as enable project leads to be successful without feeling discouraged or overwhelmed. To help map out the simple process, a project pathway was created and is included in the toolkit. The project pathway helps guide a clinical nurse and other interprofessional colleagues down a clear road to project implementation. Figure 7.2 shows the six simple steps an employee needs to take to move a project from idea to implementation and ultimately to project sharing using the FLIGHT Model.

Unit Project Pathway

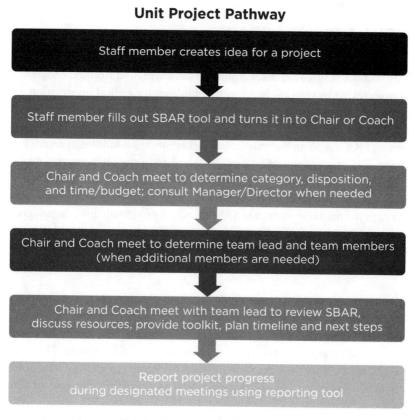

FIGURE 7.2   Project pathway.

This tool helps individuals map a project pathway and guides employees with an idea about what to do next. One goal we had when developing the FLIGHT tools was to ensure the steps and processes were as simple as possible. We knew the process needed to encourage participation and foster confidence that ideas could be put into action. We did not want a process that would be cumbersome or discouraging/overwhelming. In addition to understanding how to move their idea forward, we wanted clarity on roles and responsibilities as well as support and resources. We felt project leaders would benefit from knowing what they are accountable for as well as how the people around them can support their success and whom to turn to if they encounter a roadblock or need additional help. Having the support, the resources, the pathway, and the tools gives all employees an idea of how to get started.

FLIGHT Tool 1: The SBAR

The starting point for any project idea within the FLIGHT Model is the SBAR. SBAR stands for Situation, Background, Assessment, and Recommendation and was created by the U.S. Navy to standardize how critical information gets communicated from one person to another, regardless of rank (Narayan, 2013). Communication errors have been an ongoing focus of The Joint Commission (TJC) due to an increase in sentinel events from failures in communication. TJC has endorsed SBAR as the template to communicate patient information at shift hand-off and interprofessional communication (Stewart, 2016). With the increased focus on patient safety and preventable harm caused from gaps in communication, the SBAR is now a commonly used communication tool in healthcare. Many organizations use SBAR not only for shift hand-off and patient status communication, but to internally communicate ideas for improvement.

Within the FLIGHT Model, the SBAR is a method for employees to marry their identified issue with an improvement idea. Because this commonly used tool in healthcare is an easy and familiar way for nurses to organize their thoughts and ideas, it can take as little as two minutes to complete. The FLIGHT Model SBAR is expanded and asks employees to identify stakeholders who may be affected by the change as well as any other colleagues or team members who may be interested in working on this project. When the SBAR is completed, the employee submits the completed form to the unit chair or coach. The chair and coach review the SBAR and ask clarifying questions to better understand the scale and scope of the project. Finally, the chair and coach determine the following:

- **Category:** Is it a patient satisfaction, employee satisfaction, or quality/safety project?

- **Disposition:** Is it a priority project that will be immediately active, or does it move to the queue waiting for the proper opportunity to be developed?

- **Time and budget:** How many hours are anticipated for this project?

Because it is necessary to keep leadership informed, the SBAR is shared with either the manager or the director to verify it is truly a priority and to allow input or additional information to be considered (e.g., regulatory requirements, unintended consequences of the project). Figure 7.3 is the SBAR completed for the case study below.

CASE STUDY: Outpatient Infusion and Emergency Drugs

A busy outpatient infusion center (OIC) delivers a large volume of highly reactive medications. Clinical nurses in OIC need to be prepared for potential reactions to occur at any moment. When an unanticipated reaction occurs, the standard of practice is to administer immunosuppressives and antihistamines as soon as possible. When there is a delay in treatment, the patient may need to transfer to the emergency department and possibly require admission to the hospital. Time is of the essence.

One clinical nurse felt frustration with the amount of time it took to gather the necessary medications and supplies and felt there was a more efficient way to store them. Her idea was to create a reaction kit in which the medications and supplies were maintained in one portable bag, so the nurse could quickly obtain the kit and immediately go to the patient's side to begin treatment. She created an SBAR outlining the Situation, Background, Assessment, and Recommendation. She also identified that pharmacy was a stakeholder and would need to be involved with the project. She presented this SBAR to the chair and coach, the manager approved it as an active quality/safety project, and budgeted hours were set aside for the project work.

The chair and coach reviewed the budgeted hours with the project lead and helped create a project plan and timeline. The manager assisted the project lead in securing a pharmacist who would work with her on the project. The project lead was now prepared to begin the work and implement the change she envisioned.

Unit Council SBAR Tool

Unit Council is designed to assist all employees in finding solutions to problems that are identified in their everyday practice. We want to know what barriers exist, but more importantly we need your ideas on how to repair the problems. Please use this form to detail **each** part of the issue you are bringing forward and return it to your unit council chair.

Situation What is the issue/problem/idea?	**High number of highly reactive medications in the Outpatient Infusion Center**
Background: What is the clinical context, hospital policy, or standard of practice surrounding the issue?	**Standard of practice is to medicate with immunosuppressive and antihistamine medications to alleviate reactions**
Assessment: What do you think the problem is? What is really happening?	**Time is of the essence in treating these reactions. The sooner the patient is medicated, the sooner the reaction is hopefully halted, thereby increasing patient safety and possibly alleviating ER admission and/or hospital admission.**
Recommendation: What would you do to correct/improve this? How might you measure the outcome? Are the proposed changes feasible and sustainable?	**In the past it has been necessary to retrieve medications from the Pyxis and gather supplies independently, which can be chaotic and costly in terms of time. A "reaction kit" with all supplies needed, including possible medications, can be assembled so the patient can be treated ASAP.**

Who are identified stakeholders who might be affected by this change?

Any patient who has a hypersensitivity reaction. Pharmacy for medication. Staff nurses.

Please provide a list of participants who are interested in working on a project surrounding this issue/problem: Karen Wittenburg, RN, MSN, OCN

Submitted by: _____Karen Wittenburg, RN, MSN, OCN_____   Date: _____9/14/18_____

For Unit Council Chair/Coach Use Only:

Category	☐ Patient satisfaction ☐ Staff satisfaction ☐ Quality/Safety
Disposition	☐ Priority Project – active ☐ In the queue
Time/Budget	_____ hours _____ Manager or Director approval

Send all SBAR forms to Deborah Smith.

FIGURE 7.3 Completed SBAR for OIC project.

FLIGHT Tool 2: The Reporting Tool

Creating opportunities for clear and professional communication of project progress to peers and leadership is an integral part of the FLIGHT Model. Professional governance provides clinical nurses with numerous opportunities to develop leadership skills such as organization, communication, and presentation skills. Not all clinical nurses, however, are confident in their ability to articulate a clear and concise message and may find communicating with leadership intimidating. Having a structured reporting tool can help inexperienced clinical nurses organize their thoughts, use data to show the need for improvement, articulate the barriers, and request additional support when needed. Project leads quickly learn the persuasive impact of using data to show the need for change and the outcome results, and that communicating barriers to leadership can save time and frustration. Figure 7.4 is the FLIGHT Model reporting tool. It is intended to be an easy-to-complete tool for project leads.

Gaining experience in presenting project updates in both formal and informal environments is important. Chairs, coaches, and organizational leaders should encourage project leads and team members to communicate to their peers during meetings or through other common communication venues. Communication can generate interest around the project, create buy-in to the proposed change, and potentially introduce new approaches to the issue at hand. Furthermore, sharing the work through various venues can be thought-provoking for colleagues throughout the organization. It is an opportunity to explore if the identified project is something that could be implemented in their own work environment and can plant the seed for possible spread of a successful project. Having a culture that supports innovation and sharing of ideas increases excitement and engagement and can change practices and outcomes throughout the organization.

> ### FLIGHT Team Check-In
>
> Clinical nurses who are working to make a difference want to feel supported and valued by their leadership. Leaders should keep a pulse on project progress and barriers either through check-ins or by being available to answer questions and talk through barriers. Project leads feel supported when a barrier exists and a leader steps forward to explore ways of removing the barrier or helps steer a project lead to a resource. Not only does the clinical nurse feel supported, but the leader shows, through individual actions, that he or she values the project and believes in the professional governance structure.

Unit Council SBAR Tool

Unit Council is designed to assist all employees in finding solutions to problems that are identified in their everyday practice. We want to know what barriers exist, but more importantly we need your ideas on how to repair the problems. Please use this form to detail **each** part of the issue you are bringing forward and return it to your unit council chair.

Situation What is the issue/problem/idea?	
Background: What is the clinical context, hospital policy, or standard of practice surrounding the issue?	
Assessment: What do you think the problem is? What is really happening?	
Recommendation: What would you do to correct/improve this? How might you measure the outcome? Are the proposed changes feasible and sustainable?	

Who are identified stakeholders who might be affected by this change?

Please provide a list of participants who are interested in working on a project surrounding this issue/problem:

Submitted by: _____   Date: _____

For Unit Council Chair/Coach Use Only:

Category	☐ Patient satisfaction ☐ Staff satisfaction ☐ Quality/Safety
Disposition	☐ Priority Project – active ☐ In the queue
Time/Budget	_____ hours _____Manager or Director approval

Send all SBAR forms to Deborah Smith.

FIGURE 7.4   Unit council reporting tool.

The OIC clinical nurse shared her project idea with her team of clinical nurses through conversations at work and in employee meetings. Quickly, her colleagues saw the value of the idea and supported its success. The OIC charge nurse supported time for the nurse to connect with pharmacy to explore potential barriers together. During the unit council leaders meeting, where all chairs and coaches come together and share their project work, the OIC nurse shared her project, how it aligned with organizational goals, the resources (time and money) it took to implement, the barriers she experienced with securing the medications according to hospital policy, how she overcame those barriers, and the successes the OIC experienced since the kit was implemented. Everyone in the meeting thought this was an innovative idea that improved efficiency and had great potential to influence patient outcomes. The discussion quickly turned to how a "kit" could look on their unit. In addition to sharing the idea with fellow unit council chairs and coaches, they shared the idea with a larger group of leaders, gaining additional validation that their work was innovative and added value.

FLIGHT Tool 3: Time Tracking Log

Each project has a projected amount of time and budget set aside for completion. In the FLIGHT Model, project leaders and project team members record their hours and the focus of their work. This log is shared with the chair and coach during check-ins and assists the project lead and project members in communicating what they are working on and the amount of time it is taking to complete. Having a clearly delineated amount of time helps the project team focus on the work and be as efficient as possible. Sometimes, however, projects take longer, and the volume of work can be greater than anticipated. The time tracking log can serve as a way of sharing this reality and securing additional resources to support the work. Figure 7.5 illustrates the simplicity of the time tracking log.

Unit Council Tracking Log
To be completed by project lead and project members

NAME	DATE	HOURS	PROJECT DESCRIPTION	UC CHAIR SIGN OFF (enter into Excel budget form)

Turn log in to Unit Council Chair and Coach

FIGURE 7.5   Unit council tracking log.

FLIGHT Tool 4: The Budget Log

Once the chair and coach have received the time tracking log from the project lead or team members, the time is entered into the overall unit council budget log summary sheet, and payroll processing for the employee is completed. The FLIGHT Model uses a spreadsheet to organize budgeted and actual resources. The overall budget log is a computer-based spreadsheet that is established to self-calculate as hours are entered. This allows an ongoing and accurate tally that provides the unit council chair and coach real-time awareness of unit council project hours used to date. By maintaining an up-to-date record of hours, the chair and coach can monitor budget progress as well as plan hours judiciously for upcoming projects. Figure 7.6 shows an example of a sample FLIGHT unit council hours tracking log.

Employee Name/ Project Member	Date	FLIGHT Project Hours	Project Name/ Notes	Category	Chair/ Coach Sign-Off
Nancy	7/6	3	Reaction kit	Quality/ safety	DM
Vivian	7/3	1	Employee recognition	Employee satisfaction	JM
Jason	7/10	3	Follow-up call project	Patient satisfaction	DM
Total Hours		7			

FIGURE 7.6 Sample FLIGHT unit council hours tracking log.

FLIGHT Tool 5: The Project Action Plan

Not all projects involve numerous actions and team members, but when they do, having a project action plan can help organize and keep team members on track with their to-do lists. This tool, used by healthcare project managers, is a simple and user-friendly way of capturing:

- The planned action
- The person responsible for completing the planned action
- The time frame the planned action will be completed by

Project action plans may be a new tool and skill for chairs, coaches, and project leads. As such, some level of project management training is needed to provide a basic understanding of project management concepts, such as how to organize a project, set up a timeline with milestones, and hold people accountable to their agreements and actions. See Figure 7.7 for the project action plan template used by chairs, coaches, and project leads in the FLIGHT Model.

PROJECT ACTION PLAN:				
WHAT	WHO	WHEN	WHY	NOTES

FIGURE 7.7   FLIGHT project action plan template.

CASE STUDY CONTINUATION: Outpatient Infusion and Emergency Drugs

The OIC nurse had some key actions to accomplish prior to successfully implementing the reaction kit. Actions included:

- List supplies and medications that should be included in the kit.
- Connect with pharmacy to learn their perspective, concerns, and ideas.
- Determine a secured area to store the reaction kit.
- Communicate and educate employees about the new reaction kit.
- Create a process for restocking the kit

These actions were necessary throughout the process, and when they were addressed, they could be checked off as completed. Any newly identified action item is easily added to the active list. This structure helps a busy project lead stay organized and on target to hit the necessary milestones and complete the project.

Clear Delineation of Roles and Responsibilities

The importance of role clarity is introduced in Chapter 1, with members of the interprofessional team understanding and valuing the unique role of each profession. Key qualities and expectations of the roles people play within the FLIGHT Model are outlined in Chapter 3. Having an outline of the roles and expectations is important when implementing a change and when there is a significant shift in the way things are done, like the FLIGHT Model. Whether or not you are leading a project, are a project team member, or are a director or manager supporting the project, it is important that all know what they are accountable to do. Outlining the various roles people play is an important part of the toolkit. Not only does it serve as a point of reference, but it also prevents an overlap and redundancy in responsibility.

Support and Resources

The final document in the toolkit is a list of potential resources and additional layers of support for unit council projects. The goal of all projects is to experience success, but it takes a team. Every organization has employees with experience, knowledge, or expertise in areas that can be helpful to project leads and team members. Although specific employees are named, there are experts available for consultation when applicable. For example, if a unit is working on a project focused on infection prevention, like CLABSI reduction rates, the infection prevention specialists are available to help review data, best practices, and potential interventions. Likewise, if a unit is looking at educating employees, there is a team of nursing professional development specialists or clinical educators available to help with setting objectives and exploring educational design. Finally, because the FLIGHT Model provides numerous opportunities for leadership development, there are additional online courses in the toolkit to provide an additional layer of support and training for those actively involved in their unit projects.

Toolkit Summary

Having a toolkit with easy-to-complete tools and resources provides clinical employees the necessary structure to turn ideas into reality. When this toolkit is used throughout an entire organization, a shared language of how an idea turns into a project plan and ultimately into a unit-based change is understood. This prevents individuals from trying to create an envisioned change, going rogue with their efforts, and ending up at a dead end and frustrated.

For leaders, the toolkit serves as a tremendous resource to share with employees. It can be used to guide those who come to them with ideas for improvement or change and for those who set a personal goal on their performance plans to spearhead a project for the upcoming year. Letting an employee know there is a standardized pathway, tools available for their use, and support along the way telegraphs that the organization values its employees' input and their innovative ideas to make ongoing and sustainable improvement.

The Training

Once the groundwork is complete and the details are in place, it's time to educate the chairs, coaches, and key leaders on the FLIGHT Model, the tools they can use, and new skills that will support the work. We designed a two-hour "Tools for Unit Council Success" class and recommend the course initially be offered frequently (at least four times) over a period of one month to cater to various schedules and to increase the probability of attendance. The class is designed to expose participants to:

- The FLIGHT Model and project alignment with organizational goals
- The shifting budget—moving from meetings to project work
- The reality of no more meetings
- Roles and responsibilities
- The process for putting an idea into action
- Tools and technology to support the model
- Quality and data measurement
- Project management fundamentals
- Communication and presentation skills

Not everyone embraces a change of this scope. Many unit council chairs and coaches will feel their existing council is functioning adequately in the traditional model and will struggle to buy in to a new approach. Units who have productive meetings, engaged employees, and paid time for meetings and work often feel there is no need to change. However, existing chairs and coaches, familiar and frustrated with the traditional model, are curious to learn more and want to explore an innovative way. These leaders are open to change and may be willing and able to stay in their current role and support the transition to the new FLIGHT Model. Unit council chairs and coaches are encouraged to attend the "Tools for Unit Council Success" class as a team. Together they explore their current reality, work through the class discussions and activities, create a shared vision, and map out next steps. In addition to the chairs and the coaches, it is essential to include key leaders who may not directly be involved in the current council structure but will need to understand the transition in order to support it. These key leaders could include: unit supervisors/charge nurses, managers, directors, and nursing professional development specialists.

CASE STUDY: Lessons Learned After Implementing a "Tools for Unit Council Success" Class

In preparation for the class, the work group knew the targeted audience should be current unit council chairs and coaches. The vision was to make sure members understood the new FLIGHT Model and the important role they played in supporting the transition that would occur on their units. The chairs and coaches were a captive audience and were excited to support the move from a council with a determined number of participants to an all-inclusive, interprofessional model, where anyone can initiate, or be involved in, a change on the unit. What the task force/work group did not realize is that a key group of stakeholders were not included in the initial education. After implementation of the FLIGHT Model, there were many questions from the unit supervisors/charge nurses, managers, and even directors who had not taken the course. Questions included:

- "I know things have changed, but why don't we have a council anymore?"
- "Can you explain what's going on?"
- "I don't understand how to support the employees."

This uncertainty made it clear to the task force that the education did not hit all stakeholders, and additional classes needed to be offered to a broader audience. The task force knew it was essential that these key stakeholders understood the model, understood the tools available to their employees, and could help clinical nurses set project goals during their annual evaluations.

When we first offered the "Tools for Unit Council Success" class, many, if not all, of the audience had some exposure to the new model—but may not have had a clear understanding of what it would look like or how it could work. Many had reservations about the model's ability to help their unit and clinical employees be successful. To support buy-in and adoption, we found it helpful to provide compelling stories or evidence regarding the choice to move to the FLIGHT Model. Sharing the historical struggles of the unit councils as well as the changing healthcare environment allows others to remember the current reality and envision the future.

Flight Simulator: Historical Struggles

- Challenges with employee engagement
  - We are struggling with getting employees on board with projects or changes that are being implemented.
- Difficulty getting momentum behind a project
  - It is difficult to keep people interested, motivated, and on task when the unit council meets just quarterly.
- Challenges with project ideas
  - We get little to no input (from employees) when we put up a suggestion sheet or send out emails.

Demonstrating the power of synergy and alignment of unit-based projects with organizational priorities allows participants to envision creating meaningful change that is relevant and supports the vision of the organization. Many class participants have experienced frustrations in the traditional model and, although committed to the work, may have had a hard time experiencing success. Using the class to help validate and explain why some of these frustrations exist can be quite impactful.

"Tools for Unit Council Success" Curriculum

Teaching the Tools

Part of the "Tools for Unit Council Success" class is used to walk participants through the new tools. Chairs and coaches are asked to bring a completed SBAR of a potential future project to class. This preparatory step serves two purposes: It provides the coach and chair with the experience of completing an SBAR, and it serves as the starting point for building out a project timeline.

Other tools, like the time tracking log and the budget log, are reviewed, and electronic versions of these tools are shared.

The participants who completed an SBAR prior to class often comment on how easy it was to fill out and how it only took from two to five minutes to complete. Having a simple and easy form, like the SBAR, is inviting rather than intimidating for busy employees.

Teaching the Logic Behind "No More Meetings"

The fact there are no more meetings is a hard reality to grasp and one that needs to be repeated and clarified throughout the training—and even through-out the first year of implementation. Because all employees are the "council" and there is no longer a representative team that routinely meets, there are no more formal meetings. Instead of formal meetings, there may be brief meetings that range in length of time. For example, an hour may need to be set aside for the project lead, chair, and coach to review a new SBAR and map out the proj-ect budget and project action steps. Setting time aside for this important work is a necessary foundation for the project. Brief meetings, conversations during the workday, or an exchange of emails and text messages can also occur to communicate project progress, ask clarifying questions, and update project team members and employees on the work taking place on the unit. By not having formal meetings and working in this flexible way, employees feel they are more supported and that leadership understands the current workforce and lifestyles of employees.

Teaching the New Budget

Class participants also need training on the shifting budget and how to track budgeting hours for each project. Because the budget has shifted from meeting time to project time, there are no longer budgeted hours for meetings. Rather, a more fluid budget based on active unit projects is in play. Some chairs and coaches may have had exposure to unit budgets and have set budgeted time aside every month for unit council meetings. Other chairs and coaches may not have had this experience. The FLIGHT Model process includes a supported discussion between the coach, chair, and project lead regarding how much time is anticipated to complete the project and the number of budgeted hours necessary. If needed, the manager or director can be consulted to provide direction given the scope of the work. Conversations like this often happened behind the scenes, but in this new model, these transparent conversations occur with chairs, coaches, and project leads and allow them to gain valuable exposure to budgeting skills.

Teaching Use of Data to Measure Change

Quality improvement and the importance of using data to identify opportunities for improvement has become a common theme in healthcare. Magnet-recognized organizations use data to show the impact of interventions on patient outcomes and continually strive to improve these outcomes over time. Clinical nurses who work in Magnet organizations should be aware of their hospital trends and priorities as well as their unit metrics to continually make efforts to improve outcomes. Some clinical nurses are not able to connect data to best practices and implementation of a rapid plan, do, study, act (PDSA) cycle to implement and measure the impact of the best-practice recommendation. According to Odell (2011):

> Recent studies have demonstrated that bedside staff nurses are not regularly participating in QI activities because (a) they lack knowledge and skills; (b) they perceive barriers to implementation; or (c) healthcare agencies lack infrastructure, support, and culture necessary for success. (p. 556)

Because they are the safety net and often the last line of defense, clinical nurses have a key insight into system failures or disjointed workflows, both of which can lead to significant safety events for their patients. Schools of nursing and healthcare organizations have a powerful opportunity to educate future and experienced nurses on reviewing data, exploring best practices, designing an intervention, and determining, through the data, the impact of the intervention (Odell, 2011).

Part of our class is set aside for a presentation by a quality-focused nursing professional development specialist who maintains unit-based data on priority organizational quality initiatives. Data around falls, hospital-acquired pressure injuries (HAPIs), catheter-associated urinary tract infections (CAUTIs), and central line-associated bloodstream infections (CLABSIs) help nurses determine opportunities for improvement and show whether planned interventions are affecting outcomes. The quality presentation includes how to define the topic and goal, determining a plan for measurement, collecting and calculating the data, as well as various ways to report and present the results. The presenter's experience with and understanding of process improvement and performance metrics makes her an ideal educator and resource for employees looking to implement a change and measure outcomes.

Fundamentals of Project Management

For the most part, nurses do not learn project management skills during their undergraduate education but are often asked to be a part of a change or an improvement effort where this skill set would be beneficial. Because project management is a new concept for unit council chairs and many coaches, carving out education during this training was imperative to the successful implementation of the FLIGHT Model. The shift to a model that focuses on projects and project management (via the chair and coach) is a very different skill set from their prior focus—how to run a successful and productive unit council meeting to move council work along.

One full hour of the training was focused on such basic project management skills as:

- Creating a timeline with a clear beginning and end

- Creating key milestones

- Creating key actions and recording them on an action log to identify the planned action, the responsible person to complete the planned action, and the time frame the planned action will be completed by

Each participant came to the class with a completed SBAR, and the class was divided into small groups. Each group used sticky notes to map out the project: project milestones, actions, and target dates. The sticky notes allowed them to easily make changes on the timeline. When the participants got back to their units, they could re-create a similar timeline on their unit-based project boards to show their colleagues how the project was progressing. This simple and interactive approach proved to be appropriate for the training and skill set of the class participants. Each participant left with more confidence to oversee and support unit-based projects; use the rapid plan, do, study, act (PDSA) process; and begin to support the project ideas that are presented.

Communication and Presentation of Projects

The last part of the training is focused on tips and tricks on presenting project ideas and project progress. Communication of projects can look different depending on the situation. Having the skills to articulate a one-minute elevator speech is just as essential as being able to formally present to a large audience. Clinical nurses are not given frequent opportunities to present project work and yet often are encouraged to seek out these opportunities for professional growth. Having structured opportunities for formal and informal communication and presentations strengthens skills for clinical nurses and other project leads. The FLIGHT Model creates multiple opportunities for chairs, coaches, and project leads to share their project progress and the impact the project has had on organizational outcomes.

A nurse leader with experience in professional presentations led this portion of the training. The focus was on presentation "do's and don'ts," professional dress, the use of the project reporting tools, and PowerPoint organization. Specifics such as how many words should be on a slide in a PowerPoint presentation may be obvious to the experienced presenter, but not necessarily to a novice presenter. Furthermore, speed, tone, and volume of voice can make an impact in delivering a message. Most importantly, practicing presentations and putting this knowledge into action are truly important.

Having organizational support and opportunities/venues for presentations to peers and leaders helps build confidence and skills necessary for the future leaders of our nursing profession. To ensure continued success with change initiatives, disseminating information through various communications and presentation modalities is key. Chapter 8 discusses various project sharing techniques to help amplify the success sharing of each project across a broader audience.

References

Joseph, M. L., & Bogue R. J. (2018). C-Suite roles and competencies to support a culture of shared governance and empowerment. *The Journal of Nursing Administration, 48*(7/8), 395–399. doi: 10.1097/NNA.0000000000000635

Narayan, M. C. (2013). Using SBAR communications in efforts to prevent patient rehospitalizations. *Home Healthcare Nurse, 31*(31), 504–517. doi: 10.1097/NHH.0b013e3182a87711

Odell, E. (2011). Teaching quality improvement to the next generation of nurses: What nurse managers can do to help. *The Journal of Nursing Administration, 41*(12), 553–557.

Saladino, L., & Gosselin, T. (2014). Budgeting nursing time to support unit-based clinical inquiry. *AACN Advanced Critical Care, 25*(3), 291–296. doi: 10.1097/NCI.0000000000000043

Stewart, K. R. (2016). *SBAR, communication, and patient safety: An integrated literature review* (Honors Thesis). Retrieved from UTC Scholar. (12-2016)

"Developing excellent COMMUNICATION skills is absolutely essential to effective leadership ... If a leader can't get a message across clearly and motivate others to act on it, then having a message doesn't even matter."

–Gilbert Amelio

8

PROJECT RESULTS: PROMOTING CHANGE THROUGH INFORMATION SHARING

OBJECTIVES

- Understand the need for proper and clear communication during any period of change
- Value the importance of project sharing and celebrating projects of all sizes

Effective Communication During Transformational Change

A fundamental element of implementing any change is communication. Buy-in increases when communication is led in a structured and supportive manner. "Both formal and informal methods can be used to disseminate information. Formal communication methods follow well-defined, systematic procedures, whereas informal communications are casual and more extemporaneous" (Harris, Roussel, Thomas, & Dearman, 2016, p. 158). Examples of informal communication include emails, texts, and social media; examples of formal communication include employee meetings, town halls, and leadership huddles. Although technology can help with communicating, it is important to acknowledge the impact of face-to-face communication.

Effective communication requires clear, detailed information to be sent and heard between the speaker and the audience. According to Heathfield (2018):

- An audience must trust the person (leader) sharing the message and be willing to listen to the message being shared.

- The delivery method must meet the needs of the speaker and audience and must be timed appropriately.

- The content must resonate on some level with the audience in order for them to connect with the message.

We recommend communicating through multiple channels to reach as many employees as possible. Some employees are visual learners and need to see what changes are occurring, while others may be auditory learners who want to hear about the changes. It is important to know your audience and communicate at the right time, in the right place, and in the right manner. Communicating in a clear and concise method targeted to your audience is essential. When planning to communicate a change to both leaders and employees, it is important to personalize the message and showcase the specific benefits both employees and leadership can experience from implementing the FLIGHT Model.

For years, organizations have grappled with employee concerns about poor communication and their desire to have clear communication on changes anticipated or occurring in the health system. They want and need a link to a broader picture. The FLIGHT Model creates and develops a communication structure that supports open discussion, leadership development, and a tiered system of support. This communication structure is the cornerstone of our model. In developing the FLIGHT Model, we embedded several methods designed to promote successful communication as well as created a system for project spread, buy-in, and support.

Effectively Communicating the Plan to Employees

When meeting with employees, successfully messaging the new approach to unit council can energize employees and highlight their widespread ability to be involved and contribute at any level. Additionally, it can help employees understand they have the ability to make a difference with employee satisfaction, patient satisfaction, and quality outcomes. This introduction is an ideal opportunity to share the organizational, division, and unit strategic plans highlighting how alignment of unit-based projects will enhance successfully reaching objectives. Furthermore, budget allocation and dedicated time for project work is a strong selling point for clinical employees—and you should emphasize this when introducing the FLIGHT Model.

FLIGHT Simulator: Benefits for Employees

The FLIGHT Model benefits employees by:

- Creating an opportunity to empower more clinical employees
- Supporting an interprofessional team approach
- Allowing for multiple individuals on a unit to participate in projects they deem important
- Allowing employees paid time to work on projects
- Allowing for creativity and innovation
- Breaking down silos and interprofessional conflict
- Allowing flexibility in work schedules to better meet work and life balance
- Tailoring to the individualized needs of off-shift workers

Effectively Communicating the Plan to Leaders

Those in leadership roles are acutely aware of the importance of benchmark data in today's current healthcare and reimbursement environment. When communicating the change to leaders, it is important to tailor the message around value stream management and the potential influence on measurable outcomes. Leaders will also appreciate the model's impact on employee engagement and employee satisfaction.

FLIGHT Simulator: Benefits for Leaders

The FLIGHT Model benefits leaders by:

- Allowing for successful and rapid completion of projects and project spread
- Assisting in managing change
- Supporting continuity, follow-through, and completion of projects
- Developing leaders at the unit level
- Increasing ownership of patient outcomes and the work environment
- Demonstrating cost effectiveness
- Increasing efficiency of processes
- Increasing enthusiasm, engagement, and buy-in

As your organization moves through the process of change, it is imperative to keep all stakeholders updated and informed of the benefits of the transformation. Communicating the message to employees will look and sound different than a message to the leadership team, but both are vital. Ongoing and consistent communication allows for a smoother transition in organizational process change.

Methods to Maintain Clear Communication

Employees and leadership both appreciate clear pathways and various methods of communication to improve knowledge of ongoing or upcoming change. The FLIGHT Model utilizes several different communication methodologies that, when used together, allow all employees to:

- Learn about the project
- Visualize a timeline
- Understand data that supports outcomes
- See opportunity for project spread

Developing a structured communication plan increases the likelihood of both system-wide and unit-level success and adoption. Figure 8.1 visually depicts the continual process and avenues of project communication.

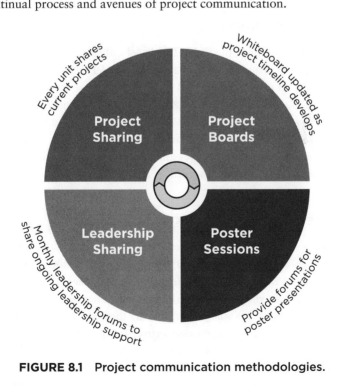

FIGURE 8.1 **Project communication methodologies.**

Communication Methodologies

As your team explores implementing communication methods into your unit-based councils, you will want to explore all of the following options:

- Use of visual project boards (whiteboards, chalkboards, poster paper)
- Project committee sharing
- Organization intranet sites
- Nursing leadership presentations
- Poster sessions

Each option provides benefits and allows teams to experience both small and large wins, building confidence and excitement for individuals.

Project Whiteboards

We suggest units that adopt the FLIGHT Model utilize a whiteboard, or other visual board, that is prominently displayed and is solely dedicated to unit-based projects. Unit council chairs and coaches should use these boards as a communication vehicle to share upcoming and ongoing projects. Project leads are responsible for updating the board on an ongoing basis (until the project is completed). The unit council chair, coach, and manager review the board and refer to the board during shift huddles and employee meetings to create unit-level awareness of ongoing improvement projects.

Committee Project Sharing

Sharing project successes and challenges with other chairs and coaches creates a wonderful opportunity for project support and spread. Is there currently a routine meeting where council chairs and coaches convene? If not, this could be a great addition to your professional governance structure. During this meeting, chairs and coaches share their projects through a traditional round-robin format. More specifically, representatives from each unit share their vision, as well as the barriers they are experiencing. Their peers can offer advice, provide support, and ask questions. After all units have shared, two to three projects are selected (complete or not) to present at an upcoming leadership forum.

Leadership Sharing Forum

Showcasing projects in front of leaders during a routine leadership forum or meeting is powerful. This is an opportunity for nursing leaders—like charge nurses, assistant managers, managers, administrative supervisors, educators, directors, assistant chief nurse officers, and chief nurse officers—to be kept abreast of the wonderful work happening on your units. During this forum, health system information can be disseminated, nursing division priorities reviewed, quality metrics plans developed, and, most importantly, two or three unit council projects are presented. Admittedly, this audience has the potential to be intimidating to clinical employees who are not accustomed to presenting. To support nurse development, we developed a standardized PowerPoint SBAR template that ensures a systematic presentation for unit council presenters. The template guides the presenter to include pertinent information (all project members, category of project, project SBAR, etc.), data collected to date, and expected outcomes. At the end of each presentation, there is an opportunity for dialogue around project support and clarification.

> ### FLIGHT Team Check-In
>
> Often, after the leadership forum, system leaders reach out to presenters to ask questions, remove barriers, and provide resources. This positive outcome has been well received by project leads and unit council chairs/coaches and is seen as an additional layer of support.

Organization Intranet Posting

As an additional method to disseminate information, we recommend creating an intranet site where unit-based projects are posted along with the name and contact number of the project lead. This facilitates an easy method for organic spread of projects. A review of projects can lead employees from other units to identify something that may work on their unit. Having a description of the project and a contact name and number allows employees to talk with one another, determine if the project will work for them, and assists in spread without re-work.

Poster Sessions

On a routine basis, we encourage holding a poster presentation day. Project leads are asked to design a poster about a project that is either in-flight or completed. The leads are asked to design their poster using information contained in their SBAR and to provide in-depth information about the project. A poster presentation day is scheduled, and the project lead or unit council chair shares his or her work with the health system. Using a large, centrally located, public room as the poster room is ideal. Unit council chairs, coaches, and project leads sign up for designated times, stand next to their posters, and answer questions. Coordinated poster sessions have proven successful as a formal method to share projects and to celebrate a unit council's success. This venue also provides employees with exposure to poster presentation skills that can be encouraged and nourished. Many unit council posters, with encouragement and mentoring, have ultimately been selected for local, regional, and even national conference presentation.

In designing the FLIGHT Model, we encourage using project boards, poster sessions, leadership sharing, and project sharing as methods for communication about project work. We recommend that adopters formulate a thorough and complete communication plan to utilize each tool provided. This plan should include creating a visual board of unit-based progress such as a whiteboard, poster boards, or magnetic boards. The goal is to keep all employees on the same page and informed. This may look different for each unit but is necessary for the success of the FLIGHT Model. Successful unit-based projects can lead to improved patient and employee outcomes. Your health system may want to develop a method to spread those projects from a single unit to multiple units or even the entire health system.

Spreading a Project Across an Organization

Sharing project work and outcomes can lead to spread and adoption across an organization. Using various venues to share identified issues, opportunities for improvement, and innovative ideas for change can increase project growth and adoption across a department and possibly even a health system. FLIGHT projects often start with one person, one problem, or a shared frustration among employees. When these pains, along with possible solutions, are shared through both informal and formal venues, other clinical nurses and their interprofessional partners often have a desire to implement the same solution to address their department needs. Anticipating potential spread is important, and efforts should be made to prevent similar projects from occurring in silos.

Instead, linking the efforts can produce a greater impact. Using a planned or strategic process to support project spread and adoption optimizes team success. Specific questions that can be used to spark robust dialogue during conversations with others regarding potential spread include:

- What were the data collection methods, or the metrics, used to determine success, and what were the outcome results?
- How was the communication plan developed, and what did it look like?
- How was essential leadership involvement determined?
- How was the team (or project members) selected?
- What is the plan for sustaining the change?
- What project feedback loops are in place?

Data Collection and Results

Using data when sharing project impact provides evidence of support for, or need for adjustment of, a plan. If a project's data demonstrate success, the small test of change can be celebrated and shared with other units. With increased alignment of projects with organizational goals, it is important to introduce data collection and measurement early in the project pathway. Without proper data measurement, it is difficult to evidence real success. It is important that members of the healthcare team participate in project management, establish evidence, and determine appropriate metrics and measurement for change outcomes (Harris et al., 2016). "As the United States healthcare delivery system is reformed, an essential lever will be measuring meaningful elements of healthcare practice to improve outcomes" (Harris et al., 2016, p. 203). Data collection is powerful and necessary in the ongoing changes of healthcare and even more powerful when proving a project to be successful and encouraging project spread elsewhere.

Communication Plans

Visualizing the plan plays an important role in the effectiveness of your communication strategy. In preparing for project spread, we recommend highlighting the benefits of spreading a project from one unit to another. Your communication strategy should ensure adequate time for discussion and questions, if necessary.

Determining Essential Leadership Involvement

When spread involves other departments, we strongly recommend that you include the formal leaders of all departments involved in your communication plan. They are essential for support and project success. Once you have formal leadership support, they do not need to be central players in the communication plan. The project team still owns the communication plan—but it can move ahead confidently knowing it has leadership support.

Appropriate Team and Project Members

An appropriate team understands the necessity for change and works together to plan and lead the identified change. This requires strong team-building, trust, and collaboration (Kotter, 2012). When communicating important aspects of the project from one team to another team, not all members of the original team need to be present; the project lead or council chair can act as the representative, provide appropriate information, field questions, and act as a resource. When we implemented the FLIGHT Model, we encouraged the project lead to be our team's representative when providing information and education at various communication venues. However, occasionally the unit council chair or another member of the team served this function. We recommend you determine as a team who will be the person to share the story and any successes realized.

Developing a Clear Plan for Sustaining the Change

After implementing the FLIGHT Model organization-wide, we witnessed variation in adoption. Some units immediately took to the new system and began projects quickly. Other units had a slower, more steady adoption pattern, starting with just one project and then moving forward as confidence in the system built. At approximately the eight-month mark, a small group of unit-based leaders met to discuss concerns about the decreasing number of unit-based projects arising from the employees. They felt that although the team was making significant strides in implementing a positive change, the team was losing momentum. This group feared the change may not be sustainable.

Sustaining a new change is a common concern of most change agent groups, large or small. Adapting from David Feeny's concept of Dolphins not Whales, Webster and Webster (2017) share a perspective on managing and sustaining change that reinforces the fact that quick wins provide a sense of positive momentum and often lead to a team's sense of achievement rather than allowing a team to focus on a single large win or success. It is natural for teams to lose momentum after an initial implementation.

Therefore, creating small wins and celebrating steps of completion will allow your team members to achieve and feel success and see their progress. Breaking a large project into many, many smaller steps—and celebrating the achievement of each step—is crucial.

Figure 8.2 visually depicts the amount of effort required to meet a delivery objective. Multiple small wins exert less effort and provide immediate gratification, whereas when attempting to tackle an entire change process at once, we expend significant effort with little opportunity to find successes. Webster and Webster (2017) suggest that this concept contributes to sustaining change.

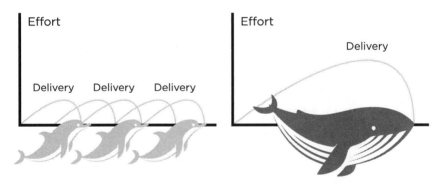

FIGURE 8.2   Dolphins not whales.
(from Webster & Webster, 2017, para. 32)

Once you have structured your project to include multiple wins, it is important to develop a consistent form of feedback with your project team and all key stakeholders.

Project Feedback Loops

We have never seen a change project effortlessly implemented. What looks perfect on paper and in theory always meets with the realities of culture, workflow, and other unforeseen roadblocks. Frequent feedback loops are imperative during project development and implementation. These checkpoints are necessary to identify possible opportunities for adjustment while considering the affected workflow. When implementing feedback loops, it is imperative to develop a structured process that supports project completion. Landau (2017) reviews concepts of project management and recommends a structured method for project status updates by using a report-out sheet. We recommend asking your project lead to come to scheduled update meetings prepared to discuss the following:

- Milestone review (planned and actual)
  - How is progress going measured against your timeline?
  - Are you meeting your milestones?
- Issues (problems, barriers, and solutions)
  - What problems or barriers is the project team running into?
    - Troubleshoot problems during this report-out or suggest additional solutions to remove barriers.
- Summary (completion date and costs)
  - Are we on time for completion?
  - Are we meeting the budgeted hours for this project?
  - Do we need to request additional resources?
- Project metrics (data, scope, and time)
  - Are we making measured progress on our planned metrics?
  - Does the scope of the project remain appropriate?
  - Do we need to adjust our timeline based on this meeting?

Project success is a team effort, and using a strategic approach will provide success to your team. Remember to keep it simple with effort and delivery, stay informed on project updates and successes, and provide support to your team using closed-loop communication techniques. Figure 8.3 depicts the closed communication cycle we recommend using when requesting project status updates. Using this structured process allows you and your project leaders to remove barriers and focus on achieving milestones, all while evaluating your metrics and budget.

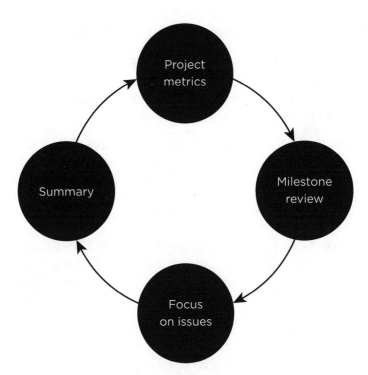

FIGURE 8.3   Project closed-loop communication cycle.

Putting It All Together: Implementing an Organization-Wide Project

Improving the Patient Experience by Introducing Purposeful Hourly Rounding

Many units had their own individual routines in place to address the practice of hourly rounding but struggled with maintaining the practice effectively. Patient experience scores reflected that the patients' needs were not being met. There were various hourly rounding log sheets demonstrating inconsistency in employees signing off that rounding had been completed.

However, employees verbally attested they rounded on their patients and often would forget to sign off on the log sheet. Employees would offer suggestions for rounding practice changes in efforts to make the process more successful, but an effective practice continued to be elusive.

The Proposed Change

A nurse on a 27-bed medical-surgical unit was sitting with a loved one hospitalized at another organization. As she provided care to her family member she became acutely aware of the benefits of hourly rounding and thought there must be a better way. As she watched caregivers care for her loved one, she noticed the hourly rounding was executed by many new faces throughout the day and night, not only by her own care team. She recognized it as hourly rounding because of the consistent script the employees utilized and decided to inquire more into the facility's hourly rounding process. Her nurse shared with her:

- The unit divided patient rooms into two groups.
- Team members signed up for time slots once or twice a shift.
- The assigned team member rounded on the assigned grouping.
- Rounding occurred with a rounding log and a standard rounding script.
- If the patient had needs that were unable to be easily addressed during rounding, the rounding team member would notify the care team members of these needs.
- Structured rounding occurred every hour during the day and every two hours at night.

The clinical nurse brought this information back to her medical-surgical floor and shared it with her unit council chair, coach, and unit-based leadership using the standardized SBAR form. The unit council chair and coach agreed the nurse should develop the hourly rounding plan as a unit council FLIGHT project.

Now that the project was approved, the clinical nurse developed a project team that consisted of three members:

- A certified nursing assistant (CNA)

- A charge nurse

- A clinical nurse

> **FLIGHT Team Check-In**
>
> This project aligns with the organization's goals to improve the patient experience and support employee engagement, thus supporting the overall strategic plan.

Using FLIGHT Tools

The team met and used the timeline, milestone, and goal-setting tool. Team members then transcribed the final tool onto the unit communication board. During shift huddles, the charge nurses shared the project purpose and goal with the entire unit while the team of three started small trials in the background.

As the project transitioned from small trials to unit-wide implementation, the team realized the larger impact they were making on the patient experience and working as a team. Purposeful rounding became a sustainable process on the unit, likely because of the successful trials and positive impact on the patient experience scores.

> **FLIGHT Team Check-In**
>
> Use FLIGHT tools to support your team's project development. Projects this big in scope will have alternate ideas or project enhancements. Allow the team to propose those ideas, but put them aside for refocus after initial success.

Using Venues to Communicate Success

Employees expressed that the process was consistently easier to accomplish and shared their new process with others who floated onto their unit. When those who floated participated in the successful hourly rounding process, they returned to their home units and talked about what they observed to their peers and leadership. After successfully implementing this new hourly rounding process on the med-surg unit, the nurse and her leadership team shared their project and data results at a monthly leadership venue during unit council project sharing agenda time. They shared the SBAR and a summary of the unit communication plan and implementation strategies. They were able to share the positive outcomes expressed by both employees and patients as well as feedback provided by the patients' families and patient satisfaction scores trending in a positive direction.

Supporting Project Spread

Some inpatient oncology unit leaders heard about the hourly rounding project at the leadership meeting. They had also recently heard about the process from one of the oncology nursing assistants who had worked a shift on the med-surg unit the week before. The nursing assistant shared that the med-surg unit's hourly rounding process seemed more supportive for the employees because each person was assigned one or two rounding times during a 12-hour shift. He shared that the employees were aware that hourly rounding was continuous, and if they were extremely focused on a higher acuity patient activity, they knew that a coworker would be checking in with their other assigned patients; this helped reduce employee anxiety during busy shifts knowing that a peer "had their back." The oncology leaders asked the nursing assistant if he would be interested in collaborating with a unit team on adopting the med-surg unit's hourly rounding routine to modify the unit's rounding needs. A project group was formed on the unit, and unit communications started in order to support the change vision strategy. The project team verbally communicated the change vision to peers at shift huddles and in unit newsletters. The messages to the employees were clear and provided details on the rounding process so all employees were aware of the expectation. Other unit communications included the project timeline on the unit council whiteboard, as well as emails from unit leaders sharing the unit council hourly rounding project updates. The project timeline posted on the council whiteboard provided a reminder for employees of the projected project

FLIGHT Team Check-In

I hear you saying, "I do not have a venue like this to invite project presenters to." Well, create one! Do you have director or manager meetings? Do you have a professional governance meeting that you can easily invite key leaders to? Find any meeting with leaders and employees together and use that venue to invite one project leader to share a project.

timeline so they could anticipate next steps and communications. The content of the communications was consistently delivered as short bullets and reminders and kept all stakeholders (leadership and employees) informed of project implementation and successes. Multiple communication venues were utilized to support the ongoing message. The project team also shared positive patient feedback on the new hourly rounding process. The project team commitment, positive patient feedback, and leadership support helped to anchor the new rounding process into the unit's culture—just as it had already been anchored into the med-surg unit.

Utilizing Poster Presentations to Support Success

To continue to the hourly rounding project story, now that two units were experiencing success it was time to share their success with others. The med-surg unit created a poster presentation at the bi-annual nursing division's unit council project sharing symposium. As viewers asked questions, the med-surg nurse sharing the poster tailored her message to the viewer. For clinical employees, she shared the effect on workflow: less interruptions from patient requests, and the general reduction in call lights overall—information supporting employee needs. When speaking to formal leaders, she would discuss the improved patient satisfaction survey results and employee satisfaction as well; this message related to the leaders' needs. The content resonated with many because the messages were tailored to the needs of both leadership and employees. The audience trusted the speaker because she had intimate experience with both the old and the newly revised hourly rounding process and could easily talk about the benefits of the change. As the sharing continued through the symposium, other employees from the project unit would engage in the conversations with their own supportive comments of the process. The excitement and passion of those involved helped engage the audience and left them wanting even more information.

Health System Project Spread

The med-surg stroke unit employees and leadership heard about the hourly rounding process at the poster presentation. They became eager to trial the process on the stroke unit. They formed an hourly rounding project group. This project group met with the oncology project employees and adjusted the rounding log sheets to the stroke unit's needs. They mapped out a project timeline and communicated the change vision and implementation to the employees. This empowered broad-based action on the unit as short-term wins were broadcasted out to all. By this time, multiple units were working on updating the hourly rounding process. The nursing division's hourly rounding process experienced both local and global communication. Local communication was within the respective units during project development and implementation. Global communication was observed as word spread to other units and among the leadership team. Effective communication delivered through multiple channels to reach a broader audience contributed to the successful implementation of hourly rounding. As the nursing division moved through the hourly rounding process change, stakeholders (employees and leadership) remained updated and informed.

Ensuring Success of Change Initiatives

Communicating change during times of transition is imperative for positive outcomes. As a leader, plan focused communication tailored to your audience (leader or employee). Suggested methods of communication include using whiteboards, project committee sharing, websites, structured presentations, and traditional poster sessions. Start with one method and build on the success of each communication method applied. Leaders should stay focused on project spread and sustaining change. Lastly, develop a system of feedback loops and focus on removing barriers while promoting the small successes with your team.

References

Harris, J. L., Roussel, L., Thomas, P. L., & Dearman, C. (2016). *Project planning and management: A guide for nurses and interprofessional teams* (2nd ed.). Burlington, MA: Jones & Bartlett Learning.

Heathfield, S. M. (2018, March 4). *How to communicate to facilitate change in employee actions.* Retrieved from https://www.thebalancecareers.com/communication-in-change-management-1917805

Kotter, J. P. (2012). *Leading change.* Boston, MA: *Harvard Business Review.*

Landau, P. (2017, August 23). The ultimate project status report checklist. Retrieved from https://www.projectmanager.com/blog/project-status-report-checklist

Webster, V., & Webster, M. (2017, April 22). How to sustain organizational change—These 5 vital ways. *Leadership Thoughts.* Retrieved from https://www.leadershipthoughts.com/sustaining-change/

APPENDIXES

A

FLIGHT UNIT PROJECT PATHWAY

Unit Project Pathway

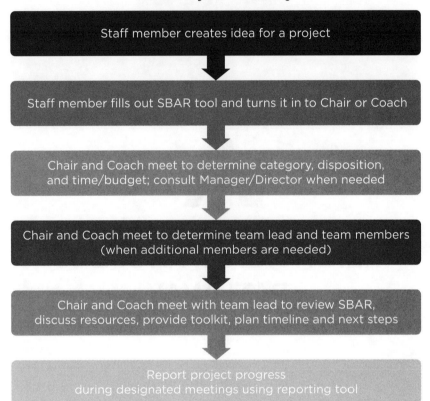

FIGURE A.1   Unit project pathway.

B

UNIT COUNCIL FLIGHT SBAR TOOL

Unit Council FLIGHT SBAR Tool

Unit Council SBAR Tool

Unit Council is designed to assist all employees in finding solutions to problems that are identified in their everyday practice. We want to know what barriers exist, but more importantly we need your ideas on how to repair the problems. Please use this form to detail **each** part of the issue you are bringing forward and return it to your unit council chair.

Situation What is the issue/problem/idea?	
Background: What is the clinical context, hospital policy, or standard of practice surrounding the issue?	
Assessment: What do you think the problem is? What is really happening?	
Recommendation: What would you do to correct/improve this? How might you measure the outcome? Are the proposed changes feasible and sustainable?	

Who are identified stakeholders who might be affected by this change?

Please provide a list of participants who are interested in working on a project surrounding this issue/problem:

Submitted by: _____   Date: _____

For Unit Council Chair/Coach Use Only:

Category	☐ Patient satisfaction ☐ Staff satisfaction ☐ Quality/Safety
Disposition	☐ Priority Project – active ☐ In the queue
Time/Budget	_____ hours _____Manager or Director approval

Send copy of all SBAR forms to nursing division administrative assistant for professional governance project sharing.

FIGURE B.1   Unit council SBAR tool.

C

UNIT COUNCIL FLIGHT REPORTING TOOL

This tool is designed to be used when communicating unit council projects to the leadership team. The intention of project reporting is to share both successes and barriers as well as to inform others of the important work occurring on your unit. When the project is complete, it's time to share!

Unit	
Project Title	
Project Lead	
Project Category	☐ Patient Satisfaction ☐ Staff Satisfaction ☐ Quality/Safety
Resources Allocated to Support Project	_____ hours
Is there data driving this change? If so, please describe baseline data.	
What is the planned change?	
What results do you hope to see? Do you have any current data to share?	
What barriers have you come up against?	
Do you need support? If so, what would be helpful?	

Submitted by: _____   **Date:** _____

When project is in process: Unit Council Chair & Coach will share update with

_____every _____

FIGURE C.1 Unit council reporting tool.

D

UNIT COUNCIL FLIGHT TRACKING LOG

The unit council tracking log is to be completed by the project lead and project members.

Name	Date	Hours	Project Description	UC Chair Sign-Off (enter into Excel budget form)

FIGURE D.1   Unit council tracking log.

E

BUDGET LOG

Employee Name/ Project member	Date	FLIGHT Project Hours	Project Name-Notes	Category	Chair/ Coach Sign-Off

FIGURE E.1 Budget log.

F

FLIGHT PROJECT ACTION PLAN

FLIGHT Project Action Plan:				
What	Who	When	Why	Notes

FIGURE F.1   Project action plan.

G

FREQUENTLY ASKED QUESTIONS

Following are questions that are frequently asked regarding the FLIGHT Model.

Q: What do your meetings look like in the new unit council structure?

A: Because all employees are the "council" and there is no longer a representative team that routinely meets, there are no more formal meetings. Removing structured formal meetings and moving toward this flexible way of connection and communication provides more support without impeding employee workflow. Specific project meetings may occur among the project team to develop and evaluate implementation. But this meeting time is limited to the support of project process.

Q: What is the difference between a chair and a project lead?

A: The *chair* remains a clinical nurse and helps to oversee all projects but is not necessarily involved in the projects. The *project lead* is any employee—a physical therapist, pharmacist, nursing aide, nurse, or secretary—who proposes an idea for change and helps lead the group in creating and implementing that idea.

Q: We are looking to redesign our partnership councils and would love to share your information with our leadership team. Can we use your same tools and data?

A: We are happy to share our tools, but it is important to know that cultural and structural components need to be in place for the tools to be successfully implemented. Please review Chapters 4 and 5 for more information on leadership and identifying areas in need of change, as this will set the groundwork for successful implementation of the FLIGHT Model. All the tools are included as appendixes as well as within the text where they are discussed.

Q: **How do we hold everyone accountable or keep track of the different projects that are taking place at the same time?**

A: Unit council chairs and coaches hold project leads accountable. Additionally, both the chair and the coach have support from their manager or director and are expected to ask for assistance when needed. Project-sharing time with leadership—in the form of various communications, including appointments, emails, or quick informal updates—is also a driver to ensure timely completion of projects. Routine check-ins and communications with leadership help demonstrate support from leadership and promote project value.

Q: **Regarding the budget, are allocated hours clerical time only and not implementation time? And are additional hours granted on top of the standard 36-hour work week?**

A: It is important to do what makes the most sense for balancing unit council work and caring for patients. There are multiple ways to reorganize a schedule to support project work. It is up to your organization to determine how to allocate these resources. Payroll and labor regulations and the need to not accrue overtime should be well understood by leaders and employees.

Q: **How are coaches and chairs elected? What criteria are used, if any?**

A: The FLIGHT Model recommends using an application process. If multiple members of a unit are interested in being unit council chair, the applications can be posted, and unit employees can be asked to elect a chair from among the applying candidates. Chair commitment is generally a two-year term, and support for an upcoming chair is done during a hand-off period. Coaches are chosen from among the unit's leadership team. It can be based on the division of labor among the leadership team, the coach's ability to be available to support the chair (i.e., coinciding shift times for curbside project management consultation), or individual interest or skill set.

Q: Our unit council handles some union contract issues like staffing plan, PTO guidelines, and unit standards. These items are not fun projects but are necessary to be reviewed and voted on annually. Does the FLIGHT Model address these union issues?

A: The FLIGHT Model does not specifically address working within a union environment. The model was created in a nonorganized, nonunion hospital. Union contract–related issues are not the focus of the FLIGHT Model; however, the FLIGHT Model could be used to further improve employee engagement and patient satisfaction. If an individual unit within a union organization wants to follow the FLIGHT Model, it will likely find success.

Q: Our organization continues to struggle with participation and engagement, and I am looking at innovative strategies to bolster our unit council but don't know where to begin.

A: The FLIGHT Model and this book will help you begin the discussion and determine what is right for your organization. Any of the authors are available, by request, for consultation.

Q: There is such a push for evidence-based practice. Do all the projects done by the unit council need to be evidence-based?

A: Not necessarily. Smaller projects may just be a simple workflow improvement measure, like our story of the fall bundle kit. The goal is to encourage employee innovation and involvement. But we recommend collecting supporting evidence for the larger projects to be able to demonstrate support or success for the project— especially projects addressing quality measures or improvements.

Q: **What if my organization doesn't have the leadership roles you describe but I want to drive change?**

A: Find a leader that you have an open relationship with and propose your ideas. Solicit the leader's feedback, guidance, and direction.

Q: **Can this model be implemented into an organization without a professional governance structure?**

A: Absolutely! Our model is an innovative way of having all employees involved in proposing ideas for change. While the structure and roles may look different, this model is a great first step in achieving meaningful change, even if your organization does not employ a formal professional governance model.

INDEX

A

abusive characteristics, 74, 75f
access to healthcare, 18
accountability, 27
  FLIGHT Model, 43
  of outcomes, 80–81
actions
  empowering broad-based, 113–114, 123
  project action plan, 141–142, 142f, 184f
adaptability, 66
adopting change, 101–117
  Bridges' Transition Model of Change, 102–103, 103f
  Kotter's Theory of Change, 105–111, 106f
  Lewin's Theory of Change Model, 104–105, 104f
Affordable Care Act (ACA), 5, 6
Agency for Healthcare Research and Quality (AHRQ), 6
American Organization of Nurse Executives (AONE), 60
analysis. *See also* evaluating
  current state, 72–73
  current state gap, 73–90
  gap analysis tool, 86t–88t
anchoring new approaches in cultures, 116–117, 124–125

B

baby boomers, 17, 17t
barriers, overcoming, 89f
Bridges, William, 101, 102–103

Bridges' Transition Model of Change, 102–103, 103f
  ending phase, 102
  neutral zone phase, 102–103
  new beginning phase, 103
broad-based action, 113–114, 123
budget logs, 140–141, 141f, 182f
budgets, 130–132, 132f
  FLIGHT Model, 42
  teaching, 148
bullying, 75f
Bureau of Labor Statistics, 7
burnout, xviii, 74

C

case studies
  anchoring new approaches in cultures, 116–117, 124–125
  communicating change visions, 111–113, 122
  comparing FLIGHT Models/unit councils, 49–51
  consolidating gains, 115–116, 124
  creating guiding coalitions, 108–110, 120–121
  developing visions and strategies, 110–111, 121
  empowering broad-based action, 113–114, 123
  establishing sense of urgency, 107–108, 119–120
  generating short-term wins, 114–115, 123
  project action plan, 142
  reporting tools, 139
  Situation/Background/Assessment/Recommendation (SBAR) reporting tool, 135

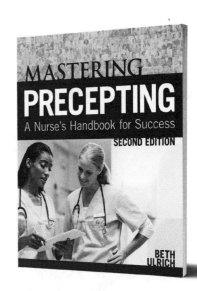
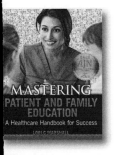
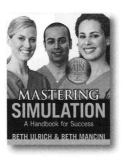
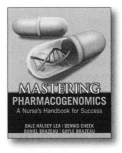
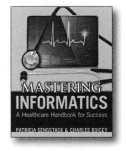
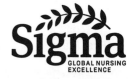

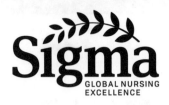
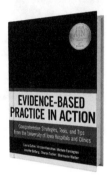
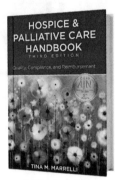
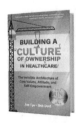
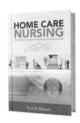
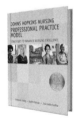
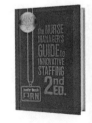